Advance Praise for

PIECES MISSING: A FAMILY'S JOURNEY OF RECOVERY FROM TRAUMATIC BRAIN INJURY

Pieces Missing: A Family's Journey of Recovery from Traumatic Brain Injury offers hope and motivation to those whose life has been disrupted by TBI. Larry Kerpelman captures the terror and ambiguity of his wife Joanie's sudden brain injury, as well as the setbacks and cumulative steps of treatment that led to her recovery. After a subdural hematoma leaves her with cognitive and physical impairments, she rallies emotional fortitude and steadfast determination to reclaim her identity, skills, and love of life. The author shares the toll that TBI takes on each family member, while illustrating how this family came together to support each other and heal Joanie. Kerpelman has a dual vantage point both as his wife's partner in crisis and rehabilitation and as a professional with a more than an average understanding of health care policy. His astute and constructive observations of the health care system will prepare families to advocate for their loved one and inform those working to improve health care.

— Janet Cromer, RN, MA, LMHC,
Author of *Professor Cromer Learns to Read:
A Couple's New Life After Brain Injury*

Pieces Missing: A Family's Journey of Recovery from Traumatic Brain Injury, is a husband's personal journal of his wife Joan's traumatic brain injury, hospitalizations, and recovery over the course of the year that followed as she is supported by outpatient rehabilitation and the care of her family and friends. Even with the advantages of being in otherwise fine health, well-educated, English-speaking, insured, and part of a caring family and responsive social fabric, Joanie and her family undergo many trials on the road to recovery. The author takes us on her journey into the pain, uncertainty, and discontinuity of TBI as well as her hospital care experience, describing an environment that is not always conducive to healing. This book is at once both inspiring and informative. It reflects their family's mutual support under difficult circumstances and joy in Joanie's recovery. As well, the author not only confirms the need for further TBI preventive efforts in the face of this silent epidemic, but also describes ways in which our health care system might improve to make experiences such as theirs more endurable.

— Jo M. Solet, PhD, OTR/L, Instructor
in Medicine, Cambridge Health Alliance
and Harvard Medical School

Larry Kerpelman has written an inspiring account of his wife Joan's hard-won triumph over a serious brain injury. By blending journal and e-mail entries with a lucid explanatory text, he draws the reader into the midst of this engrossing tale. The critical role of the Kerpelman family in Joan's recovery emerges, quite free of sentimentality, a welcome feature in the dramatic medical recovery genre. Additionally, the author makes many keen observations about the American medical care system, using Joan's experiences as telling and appropriate examples.

— Henry Vaillant, MD, Chair, Department
of Medicine, Emerson Hospital

Pieces Missing

PIECES MISSING

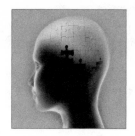

*A Family's Journey of Recovery from
Traumatic Brain Injury*

LARRY C. KERPELMAN, PH.D.

Two Harbors Press
Minneapolis, MN

Two Harbors Press
212 3rd Avenue North, Suite 290
Minneapolis, MN 55401
612.455.2293
www.TwoHarborsPress.com

Where I have used a person's real name in this book, I have done so with that person's written permission. Some people's names are pseudonyms, however, to protect their privacy. Also, at various places in this book I recreate spoken dialogue. I didn't take notes as those conversations occurred, so what is reported here is not verbatim. But it does represent the general tenor of those conversations.

Although this book contains information of a medical nature, neither the publisher nor the author is engaged in rendering professional advice or services to the individual reader. Traumatic brain injury is an umbrella rubric that subsumes a number of specific diagnoses that occur as a result of traumatic assaults to the brain, and each case is different. The information contained in this book is not intended as a substitute for consulting with your physician, whom you should consult on all matters pertaining to your health. Neither the author nor the publisher are liable or responsible for any loss, injury, or damage allegedly arising from any information, suggestions, or ideas contained in this book.

ISBN-13: 978-1-937293-06-2
LCCN: 2011931884

Distributed by Itasca Books

Cover Design and Typeset by Sophie Chi

Printed in the United States of America

To Joan, with love, again.

There is a comfort in the strength of love;
'Twill make a thing endurable, which else
Would overset the brain, or break the heart

From "Michael" by William Wordsworth

The *brain* gives the heart its sight. The
heart gives the *brain* its vision.

From "Quotations on Brain," by Rob
Kall, Futurehealth Inc., http://www.
futurehealth.org/qbrain.htm

CONTENTS

1

WAITING

THE SURGICAL INTENSIVE Care Unit's waiting
room is quiet and empty at eleven o'clock at night.
No surprise, as the only surgery one might expect to
be going on at that time of night is the relatively rare
emergency surgery. Janna, my daughter, and I settle in
to await the neurosurgeon's report on the outcome of
the surgery he and his team left just a few minutes ago
to perform on my wife Joanie.

Like the room itself, the large flat-screen television
on the wall above us is blank and silent. Neither Janna
nor I are inclined to turn it on as we wait for the
neurosurgeon to return to brief us on how the operation
went. Nor are we inclined to talk much, tired as we are
by all that has happened over the last few days to my
wife (and Janna's mother). We are both glad that the
Lahey Clinic has provided comfortable reclining chairs

for the patients' friends and families to use as their loved ones undergo or recover from surgery.

The rush of events that led us here to the surgery unit's waiting room has left us both drained. Despite that and the early morning hour, my daughter does not fall asleep. I manage to take a few catnaps while we wait, however. I awake at one o'clock, two hours to the minute that they rolled Joanie into the operating room.

At 1:05 a.m., the waiting room is still quiet and devoid of people, save Janna and me, when the neurosurgeon comes in to tell us the results of the operation.

2

INJURY

OUR WALKS BACK from the Boston Bean coffee house in Maynard always finish the same way, with Joanie pulling way ahead of me and then jogging around the corner and down the last few hundred yards to our house. But not today.

When I turn the corner, about three minutes behind her, I see my wife lying on her back on a neighbor's lawn. The street is strangely silent and still—no wind, no traffic, no sound of birds.

It is unseasonably warm for early December, so I assume Joanie is relaxing and cooling off on the grass while she waits for me to catch up. She waves her arm languorously as if to call me over, confirming my assumption—or so it seems. Then:

"Larry, I'm hurt!"

I run full speed toward her, and as I close the distance between us, I see the blood. When I get to her, my heart is racing as much from the anxiety of seeing her lying there as from the exertion of running the fifty yards to get to her. I kneel beside her. Blood is dripping from a cut near her right eye and from heavy abrasions on her lower lip, the red seeping into her hair as she lies there, face up. The sleeve of her grey sweatshirt is red, too—from where she had used it to wipe her face and hair. My first thought is that she has been struck by a car and thrown onto the lawn as she jogged down Robert Road—that's how torn and battered she appears to be. I ask her what happened.

The pain slowing her words, she answers: "My feet got caught in the laces of my sneakers, and I fell on my face onto the road. I crawled over here to get out of the road. I felt such a whack when I hit." She adds, "This can't be good."

I take out my handkerchief, wipe more of the blood away from her lip and eye, and assess the situation. She has some bad cuts and bruises on her face, but having dealt with the occasional wounds our children acquired as they were growing up, I think that these, too, will pass eventually with the application of ice and a rest.

Suspecting nothing worse, I tell her, "Wait here. I'll get the car and we'll get you home."

I run to our garage, get into my car, and reverse the two hundred yards down the street to where she is lying. Gently, gingerly, I help her into the car.

Once home, I clean her cuts and bruises. I put ice in a couple of Ziploc bags and hand them to her to put on her lip and eye, both of which are now beginning to swell. She sits at our kitchen desk as she tries to calm down.

"I'm going to look awful for Christmas," she says.

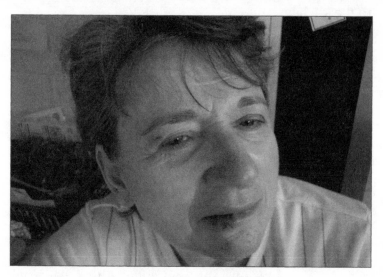

Joanie, bruised and battered, just after her accident.

Trying hard to work out a sensible plan of action, I suggest, "Well, we can wait and see what happens—see how you feel in a little while. Or we can call Acton Medical now and see what they have to say. If you feel really bad, we can go to the Emergency Room."

Acton Medical Associates, our physicians' office, is only a short ride away, but this being the weekend, there's likely to be only a skeleton staff there. We kick around possible courses of action as she sits there, but before we reach a decision, she announces, "I'm going to take a shower first, Lar. If we're going to go to Acton Medical or the ER, I'll at least wash the blood out of my hair and get into some clean clothes. Let's see how I feel after that." A hopeful sign, I think, caring about her appearance. After a shower and a short rest, she returns to the kitchen.

"Larry, you better phone Acton Medical. My head feels much worse."

The nurse on weekend duty there listens to my description of Joanie and her fall then tells me, "You should get her over to the Emergency Room at Emerson Hospital. They have equipment there we don't have at our office that would be able to tell if there's any hidden damage."

I think that is possibly an over-reaction to what appears to me to be just cuts and abrasions on her face— *bad* cuts and abrasions, sure, but not anything that won't heal with time. After all, as painful as her wounds are, Joanie is conscious, able to talk and walk, and does not seem to have any other grave injuries that I can see. We have had a few experiences in our family where a visit to the Emergency Room was called for—when our son, as a toddler, fell against a table and opened up a gash in his forehead, and when our daughter, as a teenager, injured her finger playing soccer—and the thought of spending hours waiting in the Emergency Room for my wife to be attended to doesn't appeal to either me or her. But taking to heart the nurse's comment about hidden damage, we conclude that the prudent thing to do is to go to the ER at Emerson Hospital in nearby Concord, Massachusetts. As the hospital closest to where Joanie and I live, it is the logical place for us to go in an emergency.

Ω Ω Ω

Joan sits in the dim, cramped office of the triage nurse in the Emergency Room as the nurse asks her to describe what happened so she can determine what to do with her next. I wait a few yards away in one of two chairs in the hallway outside the office while the nurse questions her and records the information she gives her. I manage to catch snippets of sentences as Joanie describes her symptoms: "achy all over from the fall," "sore wrists," "chest hurts," and "my head aches badly." The nurse records Joanie's recitation and then directs us to wait in the hospital's Urgent Care Unit across the hall.

In contrast to the old Emergency Department, the Urgent Care Unit is bright and relatively quiet. It is a new addition to Emerson's facility, having been put in only a year before to afford more space for the hospital's overall emergency operations. After giving the receptionist there identifying information and data about Joanie's insurance coverage, we wait on a couch in the Urgent Care waiting room to be called to be seen.

I tell Joanie how bad I feel for her, suffering an injury while engaging in something that was meant to contribute to her health and well-being. She expresses the same to me, and we commiserate about the irony of it all. After close to an hour of waiting, we are directed to go to a treatment room. The blood on Joanie's face has begun to clot, but her lip and eye are still noticeably swollen. As I help her to her feet, she cries out "Larry!" and then crumples. I catch her before she lands on the floor, and, seeing that she is unable to stand on her own, I hold her up and yell, "Somebody get a wheelchair. We need help here!" She seems to be conscious, but she can't stand. I begin to think this may be getting serious.

A young patient care technician appears and, between the two of us, we maneuver my wife onto a wheelchair and into a room where she transfers, with the help of the technician, to the bed. A nurse wearing a multi-floral tunic top comes in.

"I'm going to take your vital signs—blood pressure, pulse rate, temperature," she says in a warm, caring tone. "Then one of our doctors will be in to see you."

She records Joanie's vital signs and leaves us alone in the room again. We hold hands and, to try to get her mind off her pain, chit-chat idly about inconsequential things we notice about the new Urgent Care center.

Presently, an emergency room physician strides in. He introduces himself as Dr. Gert Walter and asks Joan about the circumstances of her accident.

"I was jogging, my foot got caught up in my shoelaces, and I couldn't move. I didn't have any other

place to go and fell over and hit my face on the road."
She relates this in a clear, even voice, the quaver of a few
hours ago now gone.

On the basis of her description of her fall, her
symptoms, the triage nurse's note, and a brief medical
history and examination, Dr. Walter orders a chest
X-ray and a computer tomography (CT) scan of her
head. She is wheeled to the Radiology Department to
have these done and then wheeled back to the room
in Urgent Care. While we wait alone in the treatment
room for the results of these imaging tests, Dr. Quentin
Eliason, a physician from Acton Medical Associates
who is covering at the hospital for Joanie's primary
care physician this weekend, comes in and asks about
the circumstances of her fall, how she is feeling, and
what has happened to her thus far in the hospital. Joan's
answers are much the same as she gave to the previous
physician a short time before. Dr. Eliason makes a few
notes and then departs, leaving Joan and me to wonder
what the CT scan and X-rays are going to show, what
the physicians are going to conclude, and what the next
steps are going to be. Meanwhile, my mind is ping-
ponging back and forth between wanting to believe that
this is just a matter of a few facial cuts and bruises and
fearing that it may be something more serious.

"The chest X-ray doesn't show any obvious
damage," Dr. Walter says when he returns a short
while later. "You may have cracked a rib, but small rib

fractures may not show up on X-rays. In any event, the treatment would be the same whether or not the rib has a small crack in it, or even if it were just bruised. Right now, let's just leave it alone; if the pain gets worse, then we'll decide what to do about that rib."

He leaves, and Joan and I are both relieved that her chest pain doesn't seem to be anything grave. We engage in more small talk as we wait for whatever is to happen next. In half an hour, Dr. Walter comes back again and announces, "Well, now I know why you have such a bad headache. Your CT scan shows a subdural hematoma on the left side of your brain. We'll admit you tonight and keep an eye on you."

Neither Joanie nor I are well-versed in the implications of the term "subdural hematoma," neither its consequences nor its cure. We look blankly at each other. I do know that a subdural hematoma involves bleeding in the head, but other than that global picture, I don't have many details about it at ready recall. Joanie recollected, some time later, that her main familiarity with the term up to that point came from television medical dramas, and its pronouncement always portended something bad. Dr. Walter's calm demeanor as he delivers the diagnosis doesn't belie any concern on his part, though, so I return from thinking that blood in the brain sounds terrible to thinking that maybe this isn't going to be so bad after all.

Dr. Walter then goes on to explain that Joanie fell so hard on the right side of her head that it violently pushed her brain (which lies slightly loose within its cranial chamber) against the left side of her skull, rupturing blood vessels and causing subdural bleeding at the left frontal lobe of her brain. This collection of blood (the hematoma), which he tells us will soon clot, is pressing against her brain tissue, leading to her severe head pain. She has suffered a traumatic brain injury, he goes on, and doubtless some neurons in Joanie's brain were stretched and torn as a result of her fall in addition to the torn blood vessels. When I hear his description of what has gone on inside her skull, I abandon hope that Joanie has suffered only minor damage.

We have both since come to be more familiar with what a subdural hematoma is—much more than we ever expected to be. It is an accumulation of blood from a break in a blood vessel or vessels, often leading to the collection of blood and other fluids around the brain, exerting pressure on the brain tissue and causing it to deform. The bleeding of a subdural hematoma occurs below the outermost lining of the brain, the dura mater (thus "subdural"), but external to the brain tissue itself. It is a traumatic brain injury for sure.

The National Institute of Neurological Disorders and Stroke defines a traumatic brain injury (TBI) as one where damage to the brain results from a sudden physical assault on the head. That attack to the head may result in either a closed head injury (such as occurred with actress Natasha Richardson in her fatal skiing accident in 2009) or a penetrating head injury (such as occurred from the gunshot wound sustained in 2011 by Congresswoman Gabrielle Giffords). The NINDS further refines the damage to the brain as being either focal, that is, confined to one area of the brain, or diffuse, that is, involving more than one area of the brain. Joanie's injury is a focal, closed head TBI.

An injury such as hers can cause all kinds of problems—some temporary, some permanent—due to not only the broken blood vessels but also the damage to the brain's neurons. Among these problems are head pain, confusion, lethargy, nausea, sleep disturbances, impaired attention, memory loss, speech and hearing deficits, emotional and behavioral problems, and seizures. Injuries on the left side of the brain, specifically, can impair a person's understanding of language, speaking, verbal memory, logic, sequencing of activities and thought, and control over right-sided body movements. Over the next several weeks we will see almost all of these problems play themselves out in Joanie.

Ω Ω Ω

She is admitted to Emerson Hospital at eight o'clock in the evening with the diagnosis of subdural hematoma.

The hospital is an acute care medical center of about 175 inpatient beds serving a twenty-five-town area in the outer suburbs of Boston, Massachusetts. Wheeler 4, where my wife's semi-private room is located, is a busy place, with nursing and medical staff, patient care technicians, food service aides, and volunteers going up and down the long corridor to their assigned tasks in the patient rooms running off either side of it. Her room itself can best be described as neither bright nor cheerless. It has a utilitarian cast to it, probably typical of most hospital rooms of its age in most hospitals of its age. The wall behind each of the two hospital beds in the room contains inlets and outlets for various tubes and cables, along with a small closet in each corner for the patients' belongings. A thin curtain can be drawn around each bed for privacy—mostly just visual privacy, as we would soon find out. A television set is mounted high on the wall above the foot of each bed. In one corner of the room is a small bathroom for the patients if they are able to get out of their beds to use it.

Almost immediately, a young nurse comes in, introduces herself, asks Joanie the same questions about her accident, and takes a medical history, as Drs. Walter and Eliason had just done. I wonder to myself why the history and answers that these two physicians elicited from Joanie a short time before didn't make their way to this nurse on Wheeler 4. It is a question I would repeat to myself over the next few days as nearly every new health care provider who sees her asks the same questions and dutifully records her answers. The young nurse places an intravenous needle into the back of her new patient's hand for use in the event that they will need to put medications or other fluids through it.

I am glad that, even though she is in such deep pain, Joanie is conscious, talking, and able to tell the nurse what happened to her and to answer questions about her medical history. I am hopeful that the subdural hematoma will just resolve itself after a few days and we can return to our normal lives. At the same time, though, the implication of the words "traumatic brain injury" begins to play on me.

"Do you think we should call Janna and Todd tonight to tell them about this?" I ask Joan regarding our children. By this time, it is late into the evening. Both our children are in their thirties and living independent lives away from us. Janna, younger than her brother by a couple of years, is clever, winsome, and utterly devoted to her mother. Todd, recently married and living in California, is bright, personable, and level-headed.

"Let's at least wait until tomorrow," she answers. "It's getting kind of late, and I'm really tired, so even if Janna gets out here soon, there's not much she can do for the rest of the night. And as for Todd, let's wait and see what they tell us tomorrow about this thing before we go getting him upset 3,000 miles away from here in California."

I stay with Joanie until she settles in for the night, and then I return home.

3

RETROSPECTION

O N THE RIDE BACK home, I try to sort out all that has happened since this morning. Everything was so normal, so usual when we started out. This bright Saturday belonged in early October, I think, not early December. It was as radiant a day as we get in New England, the sun shining down, the air clear and crisp as a fall apple. We have done this three-mile morning walk so many times, Joanie and I, we probably could do it with our eyes closed. Yet today's walk turned out so differently from all the others we've done before.

We've been walking regularly from our home in Acton to Maynard, the next town over, to have breakfast at the Boston Bean House ever since it opened ten years before. As we'd stride to our destination, we'd usually remark on the happenings and people along our route. The banter earlier today was as mundane as usual:

"That house over by the town line is for sale."

"Didn't they just buy it less than two years ago? I wonder if someone there lost his job."

"Hey, look. That looks like Sonya and her baby jogging along toward us at the bottom of the hill."

"Maybe we'll get to see her and the baby before they turn in to their house."

We had come to be acquainted with Sonya and her husband from waving to them as we regularly walked by their house on our way to the coffee shop. One day we noticed balloons attached to their mailbox heralding the birth of a baby boy. The next day, we attached a new-baby card to their mailbox, signing it "Joanie and Larry Kerpelman, the walkers from Acton." Ever since, we would stop and chat whenever we passed one another during our walks. Sonya often jogged "our" route, pushing along a three-wheeled child jogger in which her infant son, Sam, was ensconced.

On today's walk, we waved to John, the Maynard letter carrier, who has been working his route at least as long as we have been walking ours. Still a little further on we stopped to look at a house that was being repaired after a roof fire. The day of the fire, a month before, we were walking by that house and, along with a small crowd that had begun to gather, we watched the firefighters as they tore open the roof to get to the base of the flames. Each time we'd pass the house since, we'd mark the progress of the repairs, which seemed to be taking agonizingly long to complete. "Looks like all they have to do now is put some more shingles on the roof and paint the siding and it'll be back to the way it was before," Joanie commented.

Ω Ω Ω

Maynard is a small town—not just in area and population, but also in its feel. Streets around its center slope down toward the Assabet River, which runs through it and which once powered the mills that were the town's reason for being in the late nineteenth and early twentieth centuries. Those streets are lined with what used to be the homes of the mill's owners, managers, and workers. The still-standing, huge nineteenth century mill complex in the center of town was once a woolen mill, powered by water from the Assabet flowing alongside it. Originally, the mill manufactured carpet yarn and carpets. After the carpet industry left the region to move south, the complex became, in the middle of the twentieth century, the world headquarters of Digital Equipment Corporation until that company was sold to, and absorbed by, Compaq Computer Corporation. Continuing its industrial evolution after Digital's departure, the mill became home to Monster.com, the large career networking Internet company, along with a number of other dot-com, high tech, and other enterprises, large and small.

Downtown Maynard consists of two streets, Main Street and Nason Street. Having resisted encroachment by big chain stores, Maynard's main shopping area retains the atmosphere of a 1940s downtown, lined with small, locally owned shops staffed by friendly, mostly local, people. The stores—which haven't been gussied up to look like modern commercial establishments—tell what they're about through their unpretentious names: The Paper Store, The Outdoor Store, Pizza Express. The town's straightforwardness and friendliness remind me of the way things used to be. Perhaps that is why I like walking to Maynard; it appeals to my historic and nostalgic leanings. Joanie likes it because of the town's small shops and its denizens, many of whom we've found to be unpretentious folks with an artistic bent.

Boston Bean House, our destination this morning as it has been every morning that we walk to Maynard, sits in the heart of downtown Maynard. It is a cheery, usually bustling place, its tables occupied by people chatting away or keyboarding on their laptops while they savor their food and beverages. The imposing LaMarzocco espresso machine that sits on the service counter is seldom idle. On the coral-colored wall opposite its entrance hang two large decorative ceramic wall plaques, and the shelves along the walls display tasteful decorative knick-knacks.

When we arrived this morning, I had my usual ham, egg, and cheddar on a croissant, along with a small decaf, while Joanie had a scone with a large half-regular, half-decaf, black. As we ate our breakfast and drank our coffee, we each read the current mystery novel we had selected from the coffee house's informal library. Joanie was reading a book by one of her favorite mystery-thriller authors, Jonathan Kellerman, and I was reading *Beneath the Skin* by Nicci French. As I read it, I delighted in seeing the different uses of words the British have for certain things: "trainers" for our "sneakers," "drinks party" for our "cocktail party," "removal men" for our "movers."

Between chapters of our books, we chatted with several of the many other regulars at the coffee shop whom we number among our friends—Denise, Linda, Dorothy, Ben, Dawn. Denise Shea is otherwise known as "The Hat Lady" for the fashion-forward ladies' hats she crafts at her studio in Maynard's ArtSpace. Linda Watskin and Dorothy Leland are a retired teacher and a retired psychiatric nurse, respectively, who, like us, come to Boston Bean House almost every day from their condo at the other edge of town (and who, like us, are avid Boston Red Sox fans). Ben Blum is a physics professor at a local art college who's also a talented musician. Dawn Schallhorn is co-owner, along with her husband Eli, of the Boston Bean House. The two of them have created more than a going business with their coffee house—they have created a real community of friends, so much so that on the tenth anniversary of their opening, the customers threw *them* a party at their shop, complete with a champagne toast, a card signed by the regular customers, and a photographer from the local newspaper to record the event. These people, along with Laura, Rob, Sander, Bill, and several others, constitute the group of interesting, quirky Boston Bean House regulars we would see on almost a daily basis.

Joanie's librarian genes (both her parents had worked at the Dean College library in Franklin, Massachusetts when she was growing up) manifested themselves several years back when she saw the books on the bookshelves at "the Bean" (as most of the regulars call it) scattered about in disarray. She took to putting them back in alphabetical order by author and then periodically repeated her efforts whenever the other customers got them scrambled again.

Today, our breakfast and reading finished, Joan took it on herself to tidy up the books before we set out on our walk back home—and on to the disaster that would throw our family into a crisis like we have never experienced.

Ω Ω Ω

By the time my short drive home from the hospital is finished, I am tired both physically and mentally from everything that has happened today. I know I won't be able to fall asleep easily. It's beginning to dawn on me that Joanie might have sustained a life-threatening injury this morning. No one at the hospital phrased it that way, but having calmed down a little by now, I've been able to recall enough about subdural hematoma from my graduate study in psychology to know that that is a possibility. This has a way of focusing my mind very, very sharply, and the thoughts that pour forth now are unsettling. Could my sweet wife, to whom I'd been married almost forty years, be in danger of losing her life? If she recovers from this traumatic brain injury, will it be only a partial recovery, and if it's that, what physical and mental capacities will she have lost? Joanie is a highly intelligent, articulate woman. We could and would engage in meaningful conversations about ideas, the world, and our life. Would all that be lost— or impaired—now that she has suffered a subdural hematoma, I wonder. After having earned a doctorate in social psychology, she turned her attention and intelligence to raising our two children and keeping our home running smoothly. How would what has befallen her affect our now-grown children? Although they were living on their own away from us, they had retained their close ties of love and respect for her. Would that now somehow be compromised?

As I sit on the sofa in our family room, I reflect, in a "life flashing before me" way, on our lives together. Until the accident, our lives were calm and even-keeled. I had retired four years earlier, although I still did a little consulting and writing in marketing communications and public relations to keep both my eye and pencil sharp and practiced. Except for a few years immediately after she received her doctorate, and a few part-time jobs, Joanie did not work outside the home. We could live comfortably, even if not luxuriously, on my salary at the consulting firm at which I worked, and we both wanted our two children to benefit from having one parent there full-time for them. Joanie volunteered, until the children graduated, in the library of the public schools our children attended in order to be near them during their formative years. As a mother, she was aware of our children's moods and idiosyncracies, anticipated and met their needs and wants, guided them sensitively through the ups and downs of growing up, loved them deeply—and loved doing all of that.

Our time since I retired was essentially our own to do with as we wanted. We traveled, visited friends, went to museums—generally enjoying the togetherness that our new leisure fostered. On November 11, a few weeks before the accident, we celebrated, as we did every year, the anniversary of our meeting each other (some forty years before), and we were beginning to think about how we would celebrate our fortieth wedding anniversary the following August.

I met Joanie the year I started as an assistant professor in the Department of Psychology at the University of Massachusetts in Amherst. I had moved to Amherst from my previous job in Chicago the summer before my first semester there was to begin. Twenty-seven and single, I had made plans to travel around Europe before I started my new post. In the middle of the summer, I flew to Moscow, Russia, where I was to deliver a paper at an international congress of psychology. It was the height of the Cold War, and I was curious to see up close how our "enemy" lived. My parents and grandparents had emigrated from what was then greater Russia in the early part of the twentieth century, so it was a thrill to be in the land of my ancestors (even though Moscow was a long distance from the part of Russia they came from). Moreover, I had arranged to buy a car at the factory in Sweden while in Europe, the first new car I ever owned up to that time (a Volvo 1800S sports car). As special as that trip to Europe was for me, on my return to Amherst in the fall to begin my teaching duties, the rest of the year would turn out to be even more special.

Several weeks into the new semester, one of my faculty colleagues stopped me in the hallway. "I hear you're planning to go to the New England Psychological Association conference in November."

"Yeah, I'm driving in to Boston over the Veterans Day weekend for it. Why—you want a ride in?"

"No, I'm not going to the conference," Sam replied. "I'm trying to arrange a ride for one of my advisees. Each psych department in New England was asked to name its most outstanding undergraduate major for an award at the NEPA annual meeting, and our department named my advisee. There's just one hitch: the kid doesn't want to go to receive the award unless the department arranges transportation in to Boston [eighty miles away]. It's an honor for the student to get this award—for our department, too—so we're kind of stuck. Would you be willing to take a passenger?"

My new little sports car could accommodate two comfortably, and I had been planning to drive in alone, so I answered Sam without much hesitation, "Sure, I can take a passenger. Who is he?"

"*His* name is Joan Paksarian," Sam smiled. "Here's how to reach her," and he gave me her contact information.

That night I called the telephone number Sam had given me for this bright senior so as to arrange when and where to meet for her ride to Boston. She groaned audibly when I told her I'd be leaving at six thirty on the morning of the conference's first day, November 11, so as to arrive in Boston in time for the opening session.

On the appointed early morning, I drove to the spot outside her dormitory where we had arranged to meet, and my passenger approached the car. She was petite and well put together, I couldn't help but notice. She appeared to be barely awake and barely friendly, I also couldn't help but notice. A sneer lurked on her face, as if to emphasize to me that she didn't take kindly to being required to get up so early in the morning.

As the miles ticked by to Boston, and my passenger became more awake, we started chatting—stiffly at first, then amiably, then animatedly—as we explored each other's lives, thoughts, and attitudes within the confines of my little car. I found her to be a smart, engaging, lively young woman who readily saw through phoniness and artifice in people. I liked those qualities.

We got to the conference in time for the opening session, and I bid my passenger farewell as we went our separate ways. At the coffee break after the opening session, though, I ran into her again.

"So, what sessions are you going to next?" I asked.

"Frankly, I wasn't planning to go to another session this morning. I'm going into Cambridge and hang around Harvard Square for a while, and then I'll come back this afternoon for the award session."

"Mind if I tag along?" Being new to Massachusetts, I had never seen Boston nor its twin city across the river, Cambridge, nor the pulsing center of Cambridge, Harvard Square.

"Sure, why not?" she said, and off we went.

So engrossed were we in seeing Cambridge and getting to know one another better that morning that we lost track of time. We had to hurry back across the Charles River to the meeting hotel, arriving at the award ceremony right at the moment Joan's name was called to receive her award.

We saw each other every day after that, which involved no little pre-arranging and sneaking around. After all, she was still an undergraduate, and I was a faculty member almost seven years older than she. By April of the following year, when the deadline approached for Joanie to decide where she was going to go to graduate school, it was time to have "the talk." She had been accepted to UCLA's excellent graduate program in social psychology—but that was on the opposite coast. The thought of our spending the next four years 3,000 miles away from one another prompted me to make an awkward proposal of marriage.

"I think I love you. Don't go," I said, managing to sound both simple-minded and graceless in the same breath. I suggested that she apply to our department instead, saying I would talk to my colleagues about a last-minute application from her. She agreed to this plan.

At the next department meeting, I timorously brought up with my faculty colleagues Joan's and my situation. We had been so successful during the fall and winter keeping our romance under wraps that only her advisor and two other faculty members knew about it. Everyone else in the meeting was surprised by the news I broke.

Normally, the department liked its majors to go elsewhere for their graduate study in order to broaden their horizons and keep both the students and faculty from becoming too ingrown. But they saw the wisdom of making an exception in this case to keep one of their best majors in the department and, I suspect, one of their newest faculty members from becoming distracted and unhappy. Besides, since she would be in the social psychology graduate program, and the graduate-level courses I taught were all in the clinical psychology program, I was unlikely to have Joanie in any of my classes. So it was that UCLA lost a promising graduate student, and I gained a woman who promised to be my wife. We were married that August, and she started her graduate studies at the University of Massachusetts the following month.

After several years of marriage, our extreme weather children came along. Todd decided to be born during a raging snowstorm. Our next door neighbor, who repaired small engine equipment, saw me in my driveway that morning frantically digging my car out to leave for the hospital. He came over with one of his machines and cleared our driveway enough for us to get out on to the road for the drive to the hospital. Fortunately, just as I was about to pull out of our driveway, the town's snowplow came by, and we followed it to the town line, where, again fortunately, the snowplow from the next town came along for us to follow almost all the way to the hospital.

Janna came along during another weather extreme. It was so hot the summer she was born that I had to go out and buy, on my struggling faculty member's salary, a room air conditioner for our bedroom in order for mother and daughter to continue nursing in some semblance of comfort. To this day, Todd dislikes cold weather, and Janna dislikes hot weather.

In the decades since, Joanie and I have raised our two remarkable children to remarkable adulthood. We have lived for the past thirty years in Acton, about twenty-five miles outside of Boston, in a neighborhood of homes and among neighbors that we love. We were pretty healthy. All in all, we had built a good life for ourselves.

Now as empty nesters and retirees, we spent as much time as we could with our children (no grandchildren yet) and taking care of Joanie's widowed mother, who at age ninety-two had recently moved into a nursing home nearby. We were active in organizations we found gratifying—Joan with the Concord Piecemakers, a quilting guild, of which she was Membership Director, and me on the Board of Directors of the Acton Historical Society, the local society devoted to the history and preservation of our historic Massachusetts town. Joanie's hobbies were quilting (obviously), knitting, reading, and walking, which she did with a passion. Mine were history (obviously), coaxing things to grow, such as a vegetable garden in the summer and

orchids all year round, and, with reluctance (in contrast
to Joanie's enthusiasm), walking and exercising to try to
keep myself in shape.

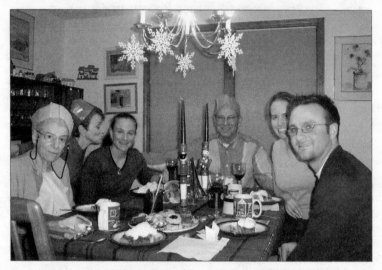

Our family before all this happened: Grandma Rose,
Joanie, Janna, Larry, Brooke, and Todd.

It was Joanie's greater enthusiasm for power walking
that put her several minutes ahead of me on our return
home earlier in the day. Joanie is petite, with short
hair and hazel eyes. Although the mother of two, she
has kept her trim, well-proportioned figure and gotten
through child-rearing with few wrinkles on her face. It
all contributes to her looking ten years younger than her
actual age. All of five feet tall (against my five feet ten),
her stride is much shorter than mine. But because she
has walked and jogged so regularly for so many years
(compared with my less zealous take on exercising), she

is able to run circles around me. This morning was no different, and I now wished I had been able to keep up with her on the last leg home. The thought of her lying there with no one to comfort her after her fall—even if it was only for a few minutes—tore at me.

Ω Ω Ω

The accident threw our family's lives out of kilter for the better part of a year. We moved sharply from "doing our thing" pretty much as we pleased to focusing on Joanie's injury and recovery. In the ensuing twelve months, we were to find ourselves spending our time in hospitals, then staying within the confines of our home while Joanie tried to regain the skills she had lost, and then cautiously going outside as Joan fought her way, literally step by step, to recovery. Yet, fortunately, her injury and its effects on her, as bad as they were, were not as bad as they could have been.

This book is based not only on my recall of what happened, but also on notes I took and e-mails I sent as events unfolded. When Joanie was first hospitalized, a nurse friend who was more familiar with the current hospital scene than I told me there would be so many people giving me information that I might not be able to keep it all straight. She suggested that I take notes, which I did, to enable me to keep clear in my mind who said what and when.

I also started sending out e-mails sporadically to our friends and relatives to apprise them of Joanie's condition. When she was getting settled into her room on Wheeler 4, Joanie recalled that we were to go out to dinner the following Tuesday with two other couples, and she instructed me to contact them.

"Tell them we probably won't be able to go," she said in superb understatement.

From my e-mails to these friends about her accident and hospitalization, word began to get around quickly, and then ever more quickly as the news spread in a widening circle. I didn't want people worrying, but I also didn't want them telephoning our house and possibly depriving us of precious sleep when we had the rare opportunity to get it, for one thing. For another, I didn't want to spend time repeating myself when answering the phone calls and e-mails I knew would start coming in once the news of Joanie's injury spread further. And last, I wanted to be sure that everyone received the same information, and that that information was well thought through, something that composing e-mails gave me the opportunity to do (while also providing me some catharsis and time to gather my thoughts).

This is my account of my wife's traumatic brain injury and its impact on our family. It's a story of how love can help overcome adversity. It's also an account of how her accident immersed us full bore into the health care system and thrust us into dealing very directly with the topic of traumatic brain injury. I didn't plan to write this book; clearly, I wish the trauma that started us on this journey had not happened at all. I began writing it because, at times throughout the whole ordeal, Joanie was unaware of what was happening to her, and I wanted her to have a record of the terrible and involving events that unfolded rapidly around her after she fell and injured her brain. I continued with it because what was happening to her revealed to me problematical aspects of our health care system, as well as information about brain injury I was not that well-versed in (despite having studied it some in the course of my graduate studies). And I wrote it to inform, and possibly help, others who, like us, may have similar challenges thrust upon them and want to know what traumatic brain injury involves, how it may affect its victim and those around him or her, how it might be avoided, and what the stages of rehabilitation from traumatic brain injury can look like. Read on and see what happens to Joanie, but bear in mind that traumatic brain injury may take forms, severity, treatments, and recovery paths different from hers.

4

HOSPITALIZATION

Sunday, December 3

THE FIRST THING in the morning, I telephone our daughter, Janna, who lives about forty-five minutes away just outside of Boston. Using the pet name Joanie and I have for her, I say, "Sweetie, Mom's had an accident and is in Emerson Hospital."

"What happened to her, and how bad is it, Dad?"

"She fell yesterday while we were walking and hit the road surface really hard. They think she has a subdural hematoma."

I answer her questions briefly as Janna questions me further about Joanie's accident and where in the hospital her mother is, but it is clear she is already on her way out the door to come to the hospital. What isn't clear, because I don't hear it over the phone, is that the news about her mother causes Janna to start crying.

Ten minutes after phoning her, I arrive at the hospital, and an hour later, Janna joins us in my wife's hospital room.

Joanie is the most important person in Janna's life. She is her confidant, her sounding board for important decisions, her rock—simply, her best friend. Joanie has always been there for Janna, and now, seeing her mother injured and inert in a hospital bed, Janna is the most distressed I've ever seen her. She stands at her mother's bedside, holds her hand, and weeps quietly.

After a few minutes, Janna asks, "Mom, how did it happen?" It's only then that I find out the details of her fall to the pavement. Until then, in the explanations I heard her give the medical people, she simply said she had gotten tangled in her shoe laces. She now gives Janna a more complete picture.

Her running shoes came with laces that were extraordinarily long—much longer than they reasonably needed to be. Indeed, when I later measured them, I found that each lace, before being tied, extended eighteen inches past the uppermost grommet of her shoe. Ever the careful person—especially when it came to her own health and safety and that of her family— Joanie habitually tied these extra-long laces on each shoe into a bow and then, because the resulting bow still flopped over the sides of her shoe, used the first bow on each shoe as she would a lace to tie it again into a second bow. This double-bowing kept the laces' extra length from hanging down the sides of her shoes. As she jogged up Robert Road on her way home yesterday, however, the second bow on her left shoe came undone, still leaving the first bow tied and her shoe still firmly around her foot (keeping her unaware that there was anything amiss). The remaining bow, now a single bow, was so large that her right foot threaded through it as she jogged along. The result: she was effectively hog-tied, unable to move her feet independently of one another, and thrown forward onto the road surface face first. It's hard to believe that this freak circumstance has led to such dire consequences.

I call our son and daughter-in-law in San Francisco, but because of the three-hour time difference they have not yet turned on their cell phones. I leave them a voice-mail message to inform them what happened and to call either Janna or me when they can. Todd telephones me a short time later. He is, of course, disturbed and immediately says, "Dad, I'll fly in to be with Mom."

"Don't make plans to come in yet," I say. "Wait and see what happens. For all any of us knows at this point, her subdural hematoma might just resolve itself quickly." Repeating what the physicians told us, I tell him, "Mom might be better and out of the hospital in a day or two."

Todd reluctantly agrees to wait until the picture clears, and I tell him I will keep him posted on how things are going. From then on, either Janna or I speak to him by telephone daily to discuss his mother's condition.

Janna decides that she will not go to work while her Mom is in the hospital. She will spend her days with Joanie and me in the hospital, she determines, and her nights back at our house in Acton, a ten-minute drive from the hospital. She makes a call to the chair of her department at the private high school just outside of Boston where she teaches mathematics to request that he get other teachers to cover her classes. He offers her no help, though, throwing the responsibility back on her shoulders to do it. On top of her distress over her mother's situation, Janna is now upset that her department chair is doing nothing to help her cover her classes. Ever the responsible one, in the evening she proceeds to make, in the middle of an already hectic and stressful situation, a number of calls to her fellow teachers to explain the situation and arrange for them to take over her classes for the foreseeable future.

As Joanie's first full day in the hospital goes on, various nurses on the floor observe and tend to her and administer medications for her severe head pain and nausea. She has eaten nothing by mouth since the accident occurred. The lines that were placed in her arms when she was admitted serve to provide fluid intravenously. Although she seems a little bewildered by the abruptness of what has happened (yesterday she was out jogging; today she is in the hospital), she talks to

Janna and me clearly and with good recognition of the
events that landed her in the hospital.

One thing I cannot help but notice about the hospital
this first day is the incredible amount of noise in it. I
expect it to be a place of quiet and repose, but it seems
to be just the opposite. Carts and beds jangle as they
are wheeled along hard- surface floors in the corridor
outside, hospital staff talk in the corridor and the nurses'
station, telephones ring, and pages are announced over
the PA system. On top of that, we can hear everything
that goes on on the other side of the so-called privacy
curtain as the other patient sharing the room is tended
to by physicians, nurses, and patient care technicians.
It is all enough to deprive an awake person of their
peace and even the best of sleepers of their sleep. And
it doesn't help that the room is right outside the nurses'
station for the floor, a center of activity. Although we
could shut the door to the room, neither Joanie nor the
other patient sharing the room wants it shut, as it then
feels too dark and isolated in the room—as if we might
all be forgotten.

Late in the evening, a patient care technician comes
in to tend to the other patient. He must have received a
page, because the next thing I know he booms out to the
nurses' station across the hall, "Tell her I'll be finished
here in a few minutes, and I'll come out to talk to her."
It was loud enough to make us jump, and had Joanie

been sleeping, I'm sure she would have been wakened with a start.

Monday, December 4

In a pattern we are to follow in the days ahead, Janna and I go to the hospital first thing in the morning to stay for the remainder of the day. On the way up to Joanie's room, Janna stops in the hospital gift shop to buy a little stuffed animal—a puppy dog—to cheer up her mother. When we get to the room and ask Joanie how she is doing, she replies, "Well, I didn't get much sleep last night. The nurses woke me every few hours to give me medicine, check on my reflexes, and ask if I knew what the date was and where I was and stuff like that."

That her sleep was broken throughout the night by nurses coming in to check her neurological signs and reflexes and administer pain medication is perhaps a necessary evil in order to monitor her condition and ameliorate her pain, but an evil that leads to a poor night's rest. She was also wakened during the night to be taken to the Radiology Department for another CT scan. I doubt that she received more than two unbroken hours of sleep, and I suspect that this is going to be the routine for all her nights in this hospital.

Despite her lack of sleep, this morning she appears to be a little stronger and better than yesterday. Although her lip and eyelid are still swollen, the color in her face is back, and her disposition is brighter. I begin to hope that this event, this accident, this trauma to her brain, will pass without much incident or long-term effect.

While Janna and I are with her in her hospital room, Joanie eats some of the soft food the hospital provides her for breakfast and drinks some of the liquids they bring her to try. At the behest of the nurses, she walks up and down the hall several times (with either Janna or me at her side to provide both moral and physical support). With both of us being with her for most of each day in the hospital, Joanie doesn't lack company. And Janna is such a sweet person that just being at her bedside helps Joanie's disposition. Her head pain and nausea continue, however.

In the afternoon, Joan vomits a copious amount of fluid and the soft solids she had been given earlier in the day—so much so that Janna has to run over to the patient sharing the room to "borrow" her plastic basin, as Joanie quickly fills up her own basin by her rapid vomiting. Some of what she throws up gets on the stuffed animal Janna had brought her, ruining it. Janna quietly takes it away.

As the day wears on, I begin to get concerned by the signs of aphasia I now see in Joanie: slowness of speech and thought, inability to find words to finish a sentence, perseveration of ideas and questions, and an occasional inability to remember the names of objects, people, and places. When I ask her, for example, what she had for breakfast, she responds, "I had some . . ."

and then her voice trails off. Asked when the last time a nurse was in to see her, she says, "It must have been, um, . . ." She cannot complete a thought nor retrieve the words needed to complete her sentences. As far as perseveration is concerned (continuation or repetition, to an exceptional degree, of a phrase or an idea), she brings up topics or phrases repeatedly, such as reminding me every half hour to call one of her friends to cancel an engagement she has with her later in the week.

The one thing she would repeat over and over in the hospital and later in the days and weeks ahead is something I can most readily understand: "Of all the stupid things to have happen to me." With all the care and caution she normally takes in her life, to have this injury befall her while she is engaging in an activity aimed at promoting her health and well-being, and to wind up in a hospital because of it, is just ridiculous and aggravating. In addition to being bewildered by what is happening to her, Joanie is frustrated and angry that it happened to her at all.

Her subdural hematoma is doing a number on her with regard to not only pain and nausea, but also lethargy and memory loss. My wife acts stunned and bewildered at times. Her speech and thought become slow as the day wears on, and she occasionally cannot recall the names of people she's known for a long time nor places we've been to often. She knows who these people are and can describe them, she knows what the places are and can talk about our association with them, but she just cannot come up with their names. There are pieces missing from her thinking.

Despite these worrying signs, a neurosurgeon's bedside visit reassures us. Dr. Quincy Edwards informs us that, if all goes well, the hematoma will be reabsorbed into her body and leave no lasting effects.

Somewhat taken aback, given how I see her condition developing, I ask him, "Will surgery be needed?"

"Not necessarily. If the bleeding doesn't progress, and the clotted blood gets reabsorbed, surgical intervention might not be needed. But as long as the clotted blood remains pressing against her brain tissue, her head pain and nausea will continue."

"Specifically, Dr. Edwards, when can those symptoms be expected to lessen, when will she get back on her feet, when will she resume normal functioning?" I pepper him in rapid-fire fashion, along with a number of other "when" questions that are very concerning to Joanie, Janna, and me. To each one, he gives what I later learn is his standard response (and probably the only realistic one) to questions of that kind: "It could be a matter of days, weeks, or months."

Imagine having a severe headache and nausea twenty-four hours a day, with the likelihood that it could last for weeks or even months. That is what Joanie is facing with this injury and might face even worse later.

Joanie receives a surprise visit from her former primary care physician, Dr. Henry Vaillant, who retired from his Acton Medical Associates practice two years before. Joanie thinks the world of him and was disheartened when he left the practice. Despite his retirement from the practice, he has maintained an appointment at Emerson Hospital as Chair of the Department of Medicine. He pops into her room, saying, "Good afternoon, young lady. I noticed your name on the list of recently admitted patients. What's that all about?"

Joanie brings him up to date on what happened and what she knows, so far, about her condition. She and Dr. Vaillant chat amiably for a while. After he leaves, Joanie comments how pleased she is that he took it upon himself to visit her.

It's not just that she likes Dr. Vaillant so much and misses him as her primary care physician. It's also that her new primary care physician of the intervening two years has so far neither visited nor called Joanie since her admission to the hospital (nor would we hear from her throughout the rest of this ordeal). I attribute this to the fact that Emerson Hospital is one of a growing number of hospitals that contracts with what are called hospitalists, specialists in the management and care of hospitalized patients. These physicians only see patients once they are in the hospital and generally don't see them either before or after. Once in a hospital, the

patient's primary care physician is not the primary care-
giver and decision-maker; rather, the hospitalist takes
over these roles.

Over the course of her three days at Emerson
Hospital, Joanie will see three different hospitalists.
The hospitalist who visits her this morning, Dr. Edwin
Inman, asks a few questions and gives us a general
overview of her medical situation. With that, he leaves
and that is the last we are to see of him.

Dr. Edwards, the neurosurgeon, arrives a little later
with more concrete details this time, telling us that
Joan's neurological signs are good, and the bleeding
of her subdural hematoma appears to have stopped.
He tells us that if a CT scan he has ordered for
tomorrow looks good—that is, the hematoma shows
signs of being reabsorbed into her body—she might not
need surgery, and she might even be discharged from
the hospital.

On top of all that has been visited upon her, Joan's
first roommate in her semi-private room, who was
quiet as a mouse, is discharged and replaced by another
woman who is, to say the least, just the opposite. The
new roommate is a young unmarried woman who
appears to be in her early thirties. She carries her body
as if problems are constantly being hurled at her and she
has to be ready to duck at any moment. Although a tall
blonde, she walks with a slight stoop, undoubtedly one
of the side effects of her many gastrointestinal ailments.

The new roommate's problems seem to span both the physical and the emotional, and she is quite vocal about expressing to her mother, who stays at her bedside, and to anyone else who visits her, how dissatisfied she is with her medical condition, the hospital, and her life.

"These damn doctors don't know what they're doing. If they did, I wouldn't be here again."

"They've got me on a liquid diet. How am I supposed to survive on that?"

"How long am I going to be here this time, Mother?"

"They couldn't do anything for me before—what makes them think they can do anything for me now?"

"Mother, why don't you just leave me alone—I'm tired of putting up with your talk."

With only a thin "privacy" curtain separating the two beds in the room, these complaints are also shared loud and clear, however non-deliberately, with Joanie, Janna, and me.

"Oh, damn," Joanie whispers to us, so as not to be overheard by the patient on the other side of the curtain, "of all the roommates to be stuck with, I have to be stranded with this roommate from hell." I am encouraged that she is showing some spunk and tingeing her comment with humor.

We take a walk in the hall, as much to get away from the roommate's rants as to give Joanie needed exercise. Joan is freer now to express her views about her new roommate.

"What is that woman's problem?" she asks. "Actually, I know what it is, and I can't really be angry at her for it—but I do wish she'd shut up and stop finding fault with everything. She has major issues with her digestive system—I understand that—but if she'd realize how her negative attitude toward her life makes things worse, she'd be so much better off. In fact, she'd likely not find herself in the hospital at all. She's just a voice beyond that thin curtain, and I'm just a vague something on the other side of it to her, so I guess we won't really be having a talk about that. But if only . . ."

Although the hospital staff had said earlier that Joanie was progressing and could be released within a day or two, by the end of the day she is not feeling all that well.

When I come home in the evening, I tap out the first of many e-mail updates I would send to our relatives and friends over the next several weeks. After writing that Joan had fallen and suffered a subdural hematoma and describing a little about what that means to her functioning, the rest of the e-mail says, in part:

> *Things have been a bit hectic, so I hope you don't mind this group status report on Joanie's condition. She is still in the hospital, but we are hopeful that she'll be coming home tomorrow (Tuesday). . . . The*

*neurosurgeon assessed her today and said that her
subdural hematoma appears to have clotted (i.e.,
stopped bleeding), her neurological signs are good, and
if a CT scan he wants to take tomorrow looks good,
then he is confident that the hematoma will eventually
disappear without the necessity of any surgical
intervention and he will release her . . . .*

*I know that you are anxious to talk to her, but
she doesn't feel much like talking on the phone and
is still not entirely "with it." She has some slight
memory deficit which, the neurosurgeon said, is likely
to be temporary—although it is expected to last a
while (weeks, maybe months—his favorite answer
to questions about the course of things). So if you
do call, I'll probably be the only one you'll talk with
(at least for the rest of this week). In fact, for the rest
of this week, I'd prefer you didn't call—it will make
things less hectic for the first few days we have Joanie
back home. I'll try to give you periodic updates by
e-mail. Her recovery from what now appears to have
been a pretty hard blow to her head when she fell
will be somewhat drawn out. She's going to have to
take things slow and easy for a while (weeks, maybe
months) until she gets back to the way she was before
her fall. But things are looking up.*

Although I'm not completely conscious of it at the
time, my reasoning for keeping concerned friends and

relatives at bay is a function of my basic understanding
of brain injury. It is not a good idea to overstimulate a
person suffering from a brain injury, and through this
e-mail and future ones, I hope to give our friends and
relatives enough information to keep them informed
about Joanie's condition while at the same time
discouraging them from trying to visit or call her and
thus overstimulate her.

Tuesday, December 5

Overnight, my wife is woken by the sounds of
gastrointestinal distress and severe diarrhea (one of her
roommate's medical problems) emanating from the
commode just on the other side of the curtain separating
her bed from her roommate's. Later that morning, after
Janna (who brings a new plush puppy for her mother
to replace the one she ruined yesterday) and I arrive,
Joan is taken down for the CT scan that we are told will
determine whether or not she will be discharged from
the hospital today. Another hospitalist, Dr. Dorothy
Quant, soon visits us to tell us that, on first look, the
CT scan appears to show no further bleeding, although
she says she will consult with other medical staff (most
likely the neurosurgeon who is following Joanie) for
more definitive word. She goes on to say that she might
discharge Joan from the hospital if her colleagues
concur and if Joan feels up to going home.

The three of us—Janna, Joanie, and I—wait to be presented with that decision, and then we wait some more. As late morning turns into mid-afternoon, Joan's roommate starts an emotional tirade that soon reaches the point of meltdown. The roommate (whom we've now officially dubbed among ourselves The Roommate from Hell) begins to complain to her very forbearing mother (whom we've dubbed The Saint) about being in the hospital again (apparently, she has been hospitalized often), about how she is being treated in the hospital, about the hospital food, and about her lot in life in general. Having by now unintentionally heard (what choice did we have?) this woman's medical history, we are sympathetic to her plight. Yet we are unsympathetic to her inability to understand how egocentric and pessimistic she is about her outlook on her problems and how that outlook, in turn, must be having a negative impact on her condition.

In particular, she rails about how she cannot get answers to questions about what is wrong with her, why she isn't being released from the hospital, and when she will be released this time. She further complains loudly that although her physician gave the okay this morning for her to be given solid food, all the hospital had given her so far was a liquid diet. We are, again, sympathetic to her plight, for we have found that in the hospital, as opposed to the outside world, definitive answers to questions and responses to requests are very, very slow in coming (often because everyone in the hospital defers to the physicians for a definitive response, and getting through to them is a time-consuming process). We've found that to be the case with even the simplest questions we ask or the simplest requests we make of the nurses: sometimes it takes hours to get a reply.

No matter how patiently The Saint explains her daughter's ills and their impact on her body to her, and how much she empathizes with her daughter about how difficult it is to get solid information about all these problems, the daughter is not mollified. She attacks her mother verbally for not understanding her, for giving the wrong answers, for just being alive. After this goes on for more than an hour, The Saint quietly leaves the room.

Some time later, a man who we assume is her primary care physician comes in to see The Roommate from Hell, no doubt prompted by the frantic pleas of her mother. As she had done with her mother, she assails this physician verbally with the same complaints and accusations. As we hear the conversation with her physician on the other side of the privacy curtain, Joanie, Janna, and I signal with our eyes to one another how serenely and competently he is handling this very difficult patient. After forty-five minutes with her, he appears to have gotten her to agree that, while she is justifiably miserable because of her many medical problems, she is making her situation worse by failing to accept how her actions are contributing to her problems.

And as to her other complaint about the food she was being served, the physician says that he will personally call the kitchen and request that they bring her solid food. At the end of the conversation, he leaves her in a much calmer state than she was in when he arrived, and we, on the other side of the curtain, enjoy a period of peace and quiet.

That lasts all of fifteen minutes. When her mother returns to the room, The Roommate from Hell starts up again, assailing The Saint with the same line of questioning and complaints as she had before. As she is doing this, a dietary aide brings her the solid food she said she longed for.

"Take it back!" she yells, "All it is is toast, tea, and an egg. I don't want it!"

By this time, the afternoon has begun to fade, and with it our hopes that Joanie might be released from the hospital today. But at last Dr. Quant, the hospitalist, appears and says that, if she feels up to it, Joanie can go home this evening, but if she'd rather stay another night, that would be preferable. We tell her we will talk about it and give the nurse our decision. Joanie, Janna, and I then confer and quickly agree that, although she still doesn't feel all that well yet, another night with The Roommate from Hell would only serve to Joanie's detriment. We tell the nurse the next time she appears that, in light of the disruption her roommate is causing, with some reluctance Joanie wants to go home today.

"Okay," the nurse replies, "I just have to tell Dr. Quant and get some paperwork together. Once we have her okay, you'll be free to go."

In a while, Dr. Quant reappears and says that she is surprised Joan does not want to wait another day before leaving, stressing that it would be better if she were to stay the night. We explain as best we can—with just the thin curtain separating us from the roommate on the other side—that all was not serene and restful in that room, and we prefer to go home where it is calmer and quieter. With some hesitation, the hospitalist accepts our decision. "Someone will be here to take out your IV," she says, "then you can get dressed."

A technician comes and begins to remove the intravenous port that was in Joan's arm, but when she does, blood begins to spurt all over Joan's hospital "jonnie" and sheets. The technician calmly puts a compress on the bleeding (the rest of us are not so calm at this point) and tells us we'll have to wait for the bleeding to stop before Joanie can be discharged.

Bleeding, lacking sleep, and impatient to leave, Joanie waits. The bleeding from her arm stops in a while, and she puts on her clothes, but she is all dressed up with no place to go. We wait, and wait, and wait some more. It seems that everything in the hospital moves at about half the pace it does in the outside world, and, after two more very long hours, the nurse finally comes in with discharge papers, prescriptions for four different medications that Joanie is to take at home, what to look for during Joanie's post-hospital recovery, and instructions for us to make a followup appointment with the neurosurgeon for two weeks from today.

We leave the hospital (a more appropriate word would be "flee") and go home. As we do, in addition to the immediate question of how long it will take Joanie to recover fully, I leave the hospital with disquieting questions that her short stay has raised about being a patient in a hospital: the noise, the lack of continuity of care that the hospitalist phenomenon seems to bring on, the joke of so-called privacy where only a thin curtain separates the two beds in the room, the medical and nursing personnel asking the same questions repeatedly. Fortunately, our family has not had much experience as patients in a hospital. Is this what hospital care is like these days?

Janna stays with us for the night at our house, planning to leave early tomorrow morning for her teaching job. I call Todd to give him the good news that his mother is out of the hospital, and I give Joanie the phone so she can talk to him herself. She does so only briefly, as she is skittish now about talking on the phone. After getting her settled in for the night, I send what will turn out to be the shortest e-mail update of the entire series:

Joanie was discharged from the hospital this evening and is now home—Yay! I'll send further details in a day or two.

Now that she is back home, I take the precaution of sleeping in another bedroom. I fear that if she and I were to sleep in the same bed, I might accidentally hit her head with my elbow and cause her hematoma to start bleeding again. But what if, I wonder, she needs help in the middle of the night for whatever reason, whether to get up to go to the bathroom or because she suddenly becomes nauseated again. With her condition so delicate, I want to have all the bases covered. To address this potential problem, I set up a signal system by moving the extension unit of our cordless phone into the bedroom I will now be occupying. I leave the base unit by the bed in our bedroom, where Joanie is to sleep, with the ringer turned off. She is to use the intercom of that phone to summon me if she needs to, and I will come running. By carrying around the extension cordless phone with me during the day, Joanie will also be able to beckon me to her bedside during the daytime.

Worried if a power failure were to happen, Janna suggests that we also place a bell by her bed that Joanie can ring to call either of us in case the intercom buzzer doesn't work. Whether by high tech or low tech means, our patient will be able to summon our help if she needs it.

Wednesday, December 6

Although no longer hospitalized, Joan continues about the same as she was in the hospital. In a pattern that will prevail for the next several days, she stays in bed most of the day wearing the old jersey and sweat pants she uses as winter pajamas. I bring breakfast and lunch (both light) to her in our bedroom, talk with her, and try to keep her spirits up in the face of her pain and nausea. As the day goes on, she becomes a little livelier, but the pain and nausea remain. I give her the prescribed codeine/acetominophen for her head pain and Compazine for her nausea. I notice that she is beginning to look (and act) more groggy and confused than she did when she was in the hospital.

A little later, though, Joan says to me, "You know, Lar, if I feel up to it, I might try to take a shower tomorrow." Although she's had sponge baths in the hospital, she has not had a shower since the day of her fall, and she sorely wants one. That she is planning one is a good sign, I think, which I place alongside the bad signs in the equation of figuring out where she stands, where this brain injury is taking her.

Janna comes to our house after her work day is over and intends to continue to do that as long as her mother is home in bed, so between the two of us we are able to take care of Joanie post-hospital. Our lives quickly assume an intense, narrow focus: Joanie and her health. Everything else seems to fall by the wayside, to be picked up in odd moments only when and if time and concentration allow. Mail, e-mail, phone messages, bills, household chores, outside meetings—we let them all accumulate. Whatever we were doing before the accident—and it's hard to remember what that was, so far have they paled into insignificance—is left by the wayside. Janna continues to do her teaching, but she makes the forty-five minute drive back to our house right after her last class each day. Normally, she would stay at school to meet with students, attend their athletic events, go to faculty meetings, mark tests, and then go home to her apartment, but she has adopted a laser focus now, too, and does only the essentials of her job so that she can concentrate on supporting her mother's recovery.

Janna and I launch into a mode of championing, pulling for, and not only being there for Joanie, but being *with* her. We don't discuss this as a plan of action—we just fall into doing it.

Our neighbors and friends offer all kinds of help. Most of them have already brought food, flowers, and gifts (in a stream that will continue for the next several weeks). For over a month, our family will have enough meals brought to us by friends and neighbors that Janna and I don't have to prepare any dinners ourselves. Now I realize why bringing meals to a household in distress has gotten entrenched as a custom: one fewer daily chore for the family to concern itself with.

Thursday, December 7

Joanie has a recurring dream. "It's the accident, all over again, Larry. I see my right foot looping into the bow on my left shoe, then falling, falling, and throwing my arms out in front of me as I try to break the fall and not being able to stop it. And then, my face hitting the asphalt and hearing a crack and then the awful, awful pain of it."

It would be a dream that, as she recovers, would find its way more and more into her waking consciousness.

A neighbor and good friend, Mary Schatz, comes over to stay with Joanie while I take Joan's ninety-two year old mother from the nursing home where she now lives to her weekly card game at the senior apartment complex where she used to live. The weekly drives Joanie or I do to take her mother to cards have become sacrosanct, as it is the highlight of my mother-in-law's week to be brought among her old friends now that she has moved to the nursing home. I don't want to alarm Joan's mother with all the details of her accident. To explain why her daughter is not picking her up today, I simply tell her that Joanie had a fall and will take a while to recover. Her mother asks a few questions, which I answer, but over the next few weeks I manage to keep the worst from her. To this day, she believes that her daughter had a bad fall that hurt her head, but she doesn't know any of the more dreadful details or how severe her injury was. At my mother-in-law's advanced age, and in her debilitated condition, the full details of her daughter's injury would only torment her and debilitate her further.

While I am gone, Joanie and Mary spend "quality time" downstairs in our family room talking. I return to find her looking better and more spirited. The wounds on her face are showing signs of healing well. There is considerably less swelling on her face than before, and the lacerations and abrasions are beginning to scab over. Things are looking up, I think.

Unbeknown to any of us, though, excess fluid is accumulating around Joanie's brain.

Friday, December 8

Joanie feels more headachy, listless, and nauseated than she did the previous two days. Her senses of taste and smell have just about disappeared, and she is highly sensitive to light. Food doesn't appeal to her, and she eats very little; talking doesn't interest her, and she talks very little. Even Janna, sitting next to her after her work day is over, cannot draw Joanie out.

Whether lying in bed or sitting up, my wife looks small and vulnerable. She looks as if she is trying to burrow into the mattress. It's at times like this that I wonder what Joanie must be thinking. Is it a replay of the fall that led to her injuring her brain, the enormity of what has happened to her, the question of when her life might get back to what it was before, the thought that she might not recover her faculties fully, the presence of the pain that has dogged her since her accident?

She expresses her frustration that she is not beginning to feel better with, "This sucks." It's a comment she makes often, all the while looking like a hurt puppy. And she repeats her mantra: "Of all the stupid things to have happen to me."

The neurosurgeon had said it would take time to recover—a matter of days, weeks, or months—so we wait and hope. It slowly dawns on us, however, that what seemed at first to be simply a hard fall onto the surface of the road while jogging—which we hope will resolve itself by the time the scabs on her lip and eye fall off—is, in fact, a serious health problem that is not righting itself, a problem, moreover, that potentially could have serious consequences. The medical people have put their best spin on the outcome of her injury, but it is becoming evident to Janna and me that their best case scenario is not necessarily what is going to happen.

My update e-mail today goes as follows:

> First, thank you all so much for your messages and expressions of love and concern for Joanie. It has meant so much to us to know that you care for her to this extent.
>
> This thing has had its ups and downs. She was somewhat animated yesterday, but last night and

tonight her head pain has been pretty bad. She is understandably frustrated that she doesn't feel better. The wounds on her face are starting to heal, but she's still generally feeling punky and headachy and doesn't feel much like eating or talking (especially today). She'll have another CT scan and see the neurosurgeon in about two weeks, and we'll get a better idea of how her subdural hematoma is doing at that point. One thing's for sure: she's going to have to take it easy a while until she's fully back to normal. Janna comes here every day after work . . . (she's sitting upstairs with Joanie right now), and between the two of us, we're taking good care of Joanie.

Saturday, December 9

Joanie remains in bed all day as pain, nausea, and listlessness continue to sweep over her. Toward the end of the afternoon, her head pain becomes so intense that Janna and I decide to take her back to the Emergency Department at Emerson Hospital, where they do a repeat CT scan to determine if the subdural bleeding is continuing. The physician attending her there is Dr. John Halporn, chief of the hospitalist service, who also may have treated Joanie while she was on Wheeler 4, but whom I had not met until now. With understated authority, he shows Janna and me the series of what are now four CT scans of Joanie's head taken at Emerson since her fall seven days ago. He points out that the bleeding has not increased from the first to the most recent CT image. Good. But he also indicates that so long as her hematoma remains (that is, is not completely reabsorbed into her body), she will continue to experience severe head pain. Not good.

He also believes that the codeine/acetaminophen she was prescribed for her pain might itself be doing her more harm than good and making Joan feel worse. He prescribes a different pain medication, Fioricet, for her, and he further recommends that Joanie's post-hospital followup appointment with Dr. Edwards, the neurosurgeon, be advanced from December 19 to the coming Monday, December 11. With the same quiet take-charge manner, he not only recommends this change of appointment date, he schedules it with Dr. Edwards himself, relieving me of one more thing to put on my "to do" list. Dr. Halporn then gives Janna and me his cell phone number and tells us to call him at any time, day or night, that we have any concerns about Joanie or if her condition worsens. I am surprised that a hospitalist is showing not only current concern for his patient but also concern for her future welfare, and I am impressed with the dedication to patient care that he shows.

I drop Joanie and Janna off at home and then go to get the prescription filled so that Joan can have the new medication this evening before she goes to sleep.

Sunday, December 10

The new medication for her head pain that she started taking last night, appears to work well—for the first twelve hours. Over the course of her first three doses of it, Joan's head pain has lessened noticeably. For some reason, however, even though we continue to give her the Fioricet every four hours, the pain relief she experienced at first has now disappeared, and, by mid-afternoon, she is back to the same intense level of head pain as before.

She lies in bed all day. Janna sits with her in our bedroom, and they watch the New England Patriots football game on television. Joan talks only a little, mostly replying vacantly and listlessly to our daughter's questions and comments. In between these sporadic exchanges, she moves her head from side to side and murmurs "Ow, ow, ow" in obvious pain. Janna tries to walk her mother around the hallway just outside our bedroom, but she can barely stand or walk. Janna calls me to come to help, and we both have to maneuver Joanie back into bed. It is clear that she is very miserable, not "with it," and barely able to stand.

In my phone call this evening to our son in San Francisco, I apprise him of these developments. I try to be realistic about the situation, struggling to keep a balance between unduly alarming him and being too optimistic.

"Dad, I'm going to fly in for Christmas," he says after listening to my report. "I don't like being out here this far from Mom while all this is happening to her."

Todd and Brooke had been married the previous summer in California and spent the previous Christmas back east with us. Their plan was to spend this Christmas in California, where her parents live.

"This was supposed to be your California Christmas," I say to Todd. "Are you sure you'd be comfortable coming in now?"

"Yeah, Dad, I am. If I fly in, Brooke will remain behind here in California to be with her parents for Christmas. I just feel so bad being so far away."

I tell him to give it more thought and then let us know his travel plans once he makes them.

5

NEUROSURGERY

Monday, December 11

THE FOLLOWUP appointment with the neurosurgeon, Dr. Edwards—the one that Dr. Halporn had arranged to move up from the nineteenth—is scheduled for this afternoon. Janna leaves early to go to her teaching job. She plans to drive back this afternoon to meet us at the neurosurgeon's office in Concord.

Joanie dozes all morning and doesn't talk much the two times she is awake. I am concerned that, in the groggy and weakened state she's been in, I might be unable all by myself to get her down the stairs from our second floor bedroom and into my car for the drive to the neurosurgeon's office. A neighbor, Judy Gettig, calls to ask about Joanie and to offer any help she can. I communicate my concern about getting her down the stairs and into the car and ask if her husband, Tom, will be around this afternoon to help. She says he will be, so I ask Judy to have him come over around two o'clock.

A little before two, I climb the stairs to get Joanie up and dressed for her appointment. I put my arms around my slumbering wife and gently try to awaken her, saying in a low voice, "Joanie, time to get up for your appointment."

"Nhmm," she moans lowly and slowly.

I try again.

"Nhmm." Yet again I try to arouse her from what I am thinking is a deep sleep.

"Come on, Joanie. Time to get dressed and go see Dr. Edwards."

Still, no words in reply, just that low moan. Putting my arms around her shoulders, I try to lift her upright, thinking that the change in position will get her going.

"Come on, babe, try to get up on your elbows." Nothing. She can't grasp her hands together around my neck, and I cannot lift her. I make a couple more attempts, each time more frantically, but I cannot rouse her or lift what is now a dead weight in my arms.

I begin to panic. I call Dr. Halporn at the cell phone number he gave me a couple of days ago to ask him what to do. When I describe the situation to him, he says, "Try even more forcefully to rouse her. I'll stay on the phone while you do."

"Wake up, Joanie! Wake up!" I shout several times at her, all the while jostling her forcefully to try to stir her. She remains completely unresponsive to my now more rapid, strenuous, and panicky attempts to get her up.

After listening to my efforts on the other end of the line for a minute, Dr. Halporn says, "We better get her to the Emergency Department at Emerson. I'll call an ambulance to take her there, then I'll call you back to let you know they're on their way." He takes down my address and phone number and hangs up.

The doorbell rings. I look out from our second-floor window to see Tom Gettig, who has come by to help. I run down the stairs and open the door.

"Tom, I can't get Joanie out of bed—she's completely unresponsive. An ambulance is coming to take her to Emerson. Wait here by the door and tell them to go to the second floor when they arrive."

As I get back to Joanie, the phone rings. It's Dr. Halporn.

"I called the Acton Fire Department ambulance; they're on their way."

By this time, however, it has already arrived, accompanied by a fire truck and a police car. Tom meets the emergency personnel at our front door, briefs them on the situation, answers some of their immediate questions, and then directs the Emergency Medical Technicians and two of the firefighters to our bedroom. Joanie is still lying inertly on the bed. One of the EMTs take Joanie's vital signs, asks her questions (to which she does not respond), and prepares to move her to the ambulance. The other EMT phones the hospital to brief them on the patient they are about to bring to the Emergency Room.

With tears in my eyes, I watch as they carry my wife of almost four decades, immobile and unresponsive, down the stairs in a carry-chair to the ambulance. At this point, I wonder if Joanie will eventually return home in worse shape than she is now leaving it, or, worse yet, if this will be the last time I see her alive. There is little time for any further thoughts, though. I pull myself together and follow the emergency responders out of the house and get into my car as they settle her into the ambulance. I yell a quick goodbye to Tom and, as I pull out of the driveway to follow the ambulance, stop briefly at the fire truck to thank the two firefighters. I have to speed up to catch the ambulance, but I do and manage to stay behind it as it makes its way to Emerson Hospital. It has its lights flashing, but it only sounds its siren once to clear the road.

On the way, I try to compose myself before I call Janna from my cell phone to give her the news. Once I give her the overall picture, we end the phone conversation so that she can get going to the hospital. Again, she arrives there in no time flat. Judy Gettig, alerted to events by Tom, meets us there as well.

Some months later Janna recalled this as " . . . the worst day of my life. When I heard Dad telling me he had to call an ambulance to take Mom to the hospital, using the word 'unresponsive' to describe her condition, I broke into tears. I just had to get to the hospital as soon as I could."

Janna, Judy, and I convene, grim-faced, at Joan's bedside in Emerson's Emergency Department while the staff on duty attend to her. She lies there, eyes closed, moving her head from side to side. The staff attending her quickly determine that Joan's blood sodium is low, a condition called hyponatremia that is often associated with a buildup of fluids in the body. It is caused, in Joanie's case, by the increased pressure on her brain from her subdural hematoma. Here's what happened. The injury to her brain that brought blood under its dura mater stimulated a defensive reaction in her body, namely, retention of extra fluid (water), which diluted her blood. This extra fluid also diluted her blood sodium level, however, which normally is within a precise and narrow range of concentration. When a person's blood sodium concentration is lowered, several problems can result. Initially, there may be confusion and lethargy. But at its extreme, hyponatremia may lead to significant alterations in mental status, such as seizures, coma, or even death. Since Joanie had been prescribed anti-seizure medication upon her discharge from Emerson Hospital a few days earlier, she avoided having a seizure, fortunately.

An Emergency Room nurse telephones Dr. Edwards at his office in the building adjacent to the hospital (where our appointment to see him today was to have taken place) to apprise him of Joanie's condition. He directs that she be taken immediately to Lahey Clinic, a large regional medical center in nearby Burlington, Massachusetts, where the main office of his practice is located and where neurosurgeons are available twenty-four hours a day. He says that once there, her care will be assumed by another neurosurgeon in his practice, Dr. Tani Nanda.

We still have not seen Dr. Edwards face-to-face during all this, so Judy calls him, urging him to come to the Emergency Department and explain in greater detail what is going on and what is going to happen to Joanie. A short time later he does, and a short time after that, Joanie is put into another ambulance for the trip to Lahey.

Janna, Judy, and I decide that, since we still don't know what we are facing here, we'll have more flexibility if we each go in our separate cars to the Lahey Clinic. In the booming, buzzing confusion surrounding this ER visit, none of us leaves at the same time the ambulance does, and we each battle the now-building rush hour traffic on our own to reach Joan's next destination. We meet, as we had prearranged while at Emerson, in the lobby of the Lahey Clinic. From there, we all go to the

Surgical Intensive Care Unit (SICU), where they've taken Joanie.

The Lahey Clinic is a 317-bed medical center encompassing a hospital, ambulatory care clinics, and physician offices. As a tertiary care center, it provides specialized medical care, usually over an extended period of time, that often involves advanced and complex procedures and treatments performed by a variety of medical specialists. Physicians in thirty-nine specialties offer services to patients, who come from all over New England and beyond.

While waiting in the SICU anteroom to get in to see Joanie, Janna makes a number of telephone calls to get her faculty colleagues to take over her classes for the rest of the week. She plans to sleep at our house while her mother is in the hospital again and spend each day with her at Lahey. I telephone Todd in California to tell him what is going on. There's no keeping him back now from seeing his mother.

"I'm going to make arrangements to come in soon," he says. "I'll let you know what they are once I make the reservations."

The SICU waiting room is busy, full of waiting relatives and friends of patients. With open pizza boxes and soda bottles on its tables and counters, it is immediately clear that families camp out in the waiting room while waiting and pulling for a loved one in surgery. Lahey Clinic has furnished this large room with an eye toward making it as comfortable as possible for the patients' families and visitors. A dozen or so well-cushioned chairs are in the room, including several that recline to an almost flat position to allow for comfortable overnight sleeping if needed. Some of the people waiting here are sleeping, covered by light blankets provided by the SICU staff. Others are watching a large flat-screen television mounted high on one wall. It is almost always on when the waiting room is occupied.

A sign next to a phone on the wall informs visitors that each time they want to see a patient they have to telephone from the waiting room to ask if it is okay to visit. If so, they are buzzed in to the unit itself, just on the other side of the door. If not, they are given an approximate time to call back. We call in and are told to call back in about half an hour, as they are still getting Joanie settled into her room. When we do, we are buzzed in to the unit itself.

Located in a brand new wing of the hospital, the Surgical Intensive Care Unit is laid out in a V-pattern, with the patient rooms—each accommodating only one patient—arrayed along each leg of the "V" and the main nurses' station placed between the two arms of the "V." Locked cabinets at the open end of the "V" hold medications and supplies. Each large patient room has three solid walls, one with a window looking to the outside and two adjacent walls separating the room

from the ones on either side of it. Each room is open
on the fourth side, exposed to the nurses' station in the
middle but fitted with a curtain that can be pulled shut
when necessary. Outside of and between every pair of
rooms is a desk with a computer keyboard and screen
where the nurses and physicians can make notes, call
up CT scans and other images for viewing, and retrieve
the patient's electronic medical record and notes. Above
each of these desks is a window with a view into the
patient room (which can be blocked by window shades
on the patient's side if the patient wants privacy). There
is a quiet urgency to the place, as patient monitors beep,
nurses and patient care technicians scurry from one
room to the other, medical and nursing staff confer,
and visitors come and go, but it all appears to be a well-
controlled urgency.

When Janna, Judy, and I get to Joanie's room, a
nurse greets us and gives us a standard orientation on
SICU's policies and procedures.

"The reason for our call-in, buzz-in system," she
tells us, "is to keep visitors out of the way when essential
procedures or care are being administered to the patient.
You should designate only one person from the family
to whom information will be given. This is to keep the
staff from having to repeat the same information over
and over as well as to guard the patient's privacy. She
can have visitors anytime, but don't have too many
people visiting her. The only time we don't allow visitors

is between seven and eight in the morning and seven and eight in the evening. At those times, the shifts change, and the day and night patient care staffs meet with each other to discuss each of the cases under their care and hand their care off to the staff on the next shift."

This orientation talk leaves me impressed with how well thought out everything is here and how accommodating they try to be with patients' families, consistent with good medical care. The SICU appears to be an extremely well-organized, well-run unit.

The nurse asks me if Joanie has a written health care proxy. I reply that she does, naming me as her proxy. She tells me to bring a copy next time I come in. This brief discussion reminds me of the possibility that Joanie may not have all the faculties necessary to make decisions for herself, and I steel myself for the decisions I may have to make for her as this crisis plays out.

Shortly after the nurse finishes her orientation talk with us, Dr. Daniel Hoit, Dr. Nanda's neurosurgery resident, meets with us briefly to tell us that the immediate plan is to raise Joanie's blood sodium level with medications, take further CT scans to check on the progress of the hematoma and the status of the excess fluid pressing against her brain, and monitor her physiological—especially her neurological—signs.

Joanie lies in the bed of her spacious private room, her eyes closed, with numerous lines in her veins and leads on her chest that have been placed there to monitor her vital signs continuously. Other lines are running into her veins to provide her with intravenous fluids and medications, most important among them the mannitol that is aimed at bringing her blood sodium level back within normal range. A catheter is in place to collect her urine. On a rolling stand beside her bed are the monitors and intravenous drip devices that the wires and tubes in her are connected to. Fluorescent-colored lines move across the monitor screens showing, real-time, her blood pressure, respiration and heart rates, blood oxygen level, and other vital signs. Around the lower part of both of Joanie's legs are flexible air-filled cuffs that alternately fill with air and then release it—this to prevent blood clots forming in her legs as she lies immobile in bed. They make a quiet "shush-click" sound as they operate.

Shush-click. Shush-click. Shush-click. Shush-click. Now with Janna, Judy, and I looking at Joanie lying there—unresponsive and with all those lines running into and out of her, the monitoring equipment letting out clicks and beeps, the leg cuff machine sounding off—questions, all unanswerable at the moment, course through my mind. Will she need neurosurgery? Surgery or not, will this pressure on her brain further impair her speech and thought? When will her intense pain end? And the most unthinkable of all, is her traumatic brain injury life-threatening?

It takes a while, but the mannitol begins to have an effect, for Joanie comes out of her semi-conscious state and stares dazedly at us. Looking at Janna, she says in a whisper, "Hi, Sweetie."

Janna grabs Joanie's hand and squeezes it. Giving her mother a warm smile, she says, "Hi, Mom. Dad, Judy, and I are all here with you." Joanie looks back at her blankly and says nothing.

Then Janna asks her, "Do you know my name?" Joanie only stares back. Janna fights back tears.

Joanie drifts in and out of sleep the rest of the day, and seeing that there is little more she can do, Judy leaves to return home. Janna and I don't want to keep Joanie from sleeping by talking to her, nor tax her when she is awake by engaging in a lot of conversation with her. When seven o'clock in the evening comes, we leave, too.

I return home exhausted by the rapid turn of events since this morning but also charged up with finding more information about all that has been thrown at us since this morning (one of my coping mechanisms). I spend some time on the Internet to find out all I can about hyponatremia, blood sodium level, mannitol, and aphasia. I also go to the Lahey Clinic's Web site for, although I have certainly heard of the institution and know its reputation, today is the first time I have been there or know someone who has. The more I know about a situation, the better able I am to cope with it.

I also feel now a stronger obligation to keep everyone apprised of the news, good or bad, about

Joanie. The e-mail update I compose tonight gives our circle of friends and family the essential details, although I still can't help but soft-pedal the more alarming ones. It says, in part:

> *This morning, Joanie became unresponsive (although still conscious, she was unable to talk, respond to commands, stand, and walk). At the Emergency Room they found that her blood sodium was low, which is correlated with not removing fluids around her brain, which resulted in pressure on her brain, which resulted in her being unable to talk or walk. If this is the problem, getting her sodium back in balance should result in a good prognosis. If that is not the case, we'll have to see where we go from there. She is in Lahey Clinic, an excellent facility in nearby Burlington, right now. Janna and I expect to be spending most of the next several days visiting her at Lahey. I don't know how long she'll be there, so I don't know when I'll have more and better information about her. But when I do, I will communicate it by e-mail. If you telephone here, we are likely not to be here, so I'm probably going to be unable to get back to you promptly.*
>
> *Once she does come out of the hospital, from all that the physicians have said, her recovery will be slow but, I hope, complete.*

Tuesday, December 12

I receive a telephone call very early from the SICU nurse who had Joanie in her care overnight. Before leaving for the hospital, I dash off an update e-mail to broadcast the good news the nurse has just given me:

> *I just received a phone call from the nurse at Lahey who indicated that Joanie is much improved over yesterday. Her sodium levels are now good, she is speaking in sentences, and she is able to identify who people are. The nurse indicates that they will likely be moving her out of intensive care today, and that she will likely be released from the hospital later this week. Much relieved, I am on my way now to visit her.*

And, indeed, I am much relieved, for the nurse made it sound like Joanie was recovering rapidly. At the hospital, Joan's mood and behavior are clearly improved from yesterday, when she could barely speak or respond to us coherently. She is more awake and can talk now, although she remains baffled and confused. She is tired from having been wakened throughout the night to have her neurological signs taken (to assess how the intracranial pressure is affecting her brain, they look for unevenness in her pupillary reflex and in arm and leg strength as well as inability to answer questions about time and place). The nurses tell us that they also sat Joanie up in a chair for a time early this morning, before Janna and I arrived, further tiring her.

Joanie is concerned and mystified about where she is. To her question of "Where am I?" we tell her she is at the Lahey Clinic in Burlington. "I don't know what that place is," she says, even though Janna and I know full well that normally she does. Then, "Is it near the Burlington Mall?" a place she knows from shopping trips made there over the years. She asks Janna and me several times during our visit to explain in detail the hospital's location, which we do. She perseverates—a sign of aphasia—on several other topics as well, which continues to worry us. And she repeats her mantra over and over again: "Of all the stupid things to have happen to me."

At home tonight, when Janna reads the e-mail I had rushed out this morning, she gets very angry at me for sending out so positive a picture of Joanie's status. Throughout Joan's hospital course, Janna has held a gloomier, but she feels more realistic, view of her mother's condition and prognosis than I have. She berates me for not giving what to her mind is a realistic picture of her mother's condition in this morning's e-mail.

"Why did you tell everybody that she was in such good shape, when she clearly is not?"

"I was simply relaying the picture that the nurse gave me in her telephone call this morning before we left for the hospital," I respond.

She is not mollified, and we argue back and forth about what I should have written in my e-mail and just how good or bad her mother's condition is.

Janna wants something definitive done to rid her mother of all the pain she is experiencing and is annoyed that, in her view, it isn't being done. And she is angry at me for not being, as she sees it, as attuned to her mother's condition as she is.

Wednesday, December 13

At seven thirty a.m., I receive a phone call from the nurse at Lahey who had cared for Joanie on the night shift. She says Joanie has improved. The details she provides sound like cause for optimism. She tells me that Joan is able to say what month, year, and day it is, and she can recall well the circumstances of her fall and a good bit of her time at home after being discharged from Emerson (although she has no memory of being brought to Lahey). She is able to complete more of her sentences, her sodium level and blood pressure are good, and she is going to be put into a chair to sit while they assess how much movement she is capable of. The nurse indicates that they will likely be moving Joan out of intensive care today or tomorrow. Much buoyed by all this positive news, Janna and I leave for the hospital to visit Joan. But this time, I don't dash off an e-mail to our friends and relatives before we go. I think it better to wait until we've at least seen Joanie.

At the SICU waiting room, we are accosted by Mary Jane, to whom we immediately give the name Queen of the Waiting Room. Mary Jane appears to be in her late twenties, a neatly dressed, dark-haired, pleasant-looking woman. She tells us she is there waiting while a relative is undergoing surgery this morning. When she spies us approaching the wall telephone in the outer waiting room to request to be let in, she asks us if we know how that process works. Before we can answer, she launches into a detailed explanation of SICU procedure: how we have to call to gain admittance, how they will buzz the door when they are ready to let us in, and a myriad of other facts about the SICU we already know.

Mary Jane then showers us with details about why she is there (her mother is to undergo triple bypass surgery), along with even more details about how her mother's need for surgery was discovered. I recognize that Mary Jane is manifesting her anxiety by demonstrating her knowledge of the ins and outs of SICU and the ins and outs of her mother's condition, but I have little patience hearing her tell me about her mother when I have my own patient to worry about. And I can see by the frustrated look on the face of my poor, tired daughter that she has even less forbearance than I have for Mary Jane. Janna practically runs in once the door is buzzed to admit us.

Arriving at Joanie's room, we find her asleep. We mention to the nurse that we have yet to meet the neurosurgeon who is principally responsible for Joanie's treatment and care. "Oh, you'll like him," she tells us. "Dr. Nanda's such a nice man. He's a favorite of the nursing staff." It is somewhat reassuring to hear that. Our friend, Judy Gettig, who is a nurse, has at times remarked that the nurses at a hospital are pretty good judges of the physicians practicing there, as they see them in both their best and worst moments.

Shortly afterward, Joanie's neurosurgeon, Dr. Tani Nanda, visits her at her bedside. He is a tall, slim man with dark black, wavy hair, a thick mustache, and a ready smile. He wears a white lab coat with his name emblazoned above the coat's left-hand pocket and the designation "Neurosurgery" embroidered just under his name. He impresses both Janna and me as a straightforward, likable person. Further, I judge him to be in his forties: old enough to have experience, yet young enough to be inclined to keep abreast of the latest advances in his field. Wary that first impressions can sometimes be misleading, I Google him when I get home in the evening and find out that he received his MD degree from Yale Medical, did his internship and residency at one of Boston's premier Harvard-affiliated teaching hospitals, and is board-certified in neurological surgery (surgery involving the brain, spinal cord, or peripheral nerves). This information about him reassures me that Joanie is in good hands with Dr. Nanda.

The neurosurgeon discusses Joanie's situation briefly but clearly with Janna and me and leaves us with the impression that the night nurse's comment that Joanie "had improved" might better have been expressed as "she is improving." He wants to keep her in the Surgical Intensive Care Unit for at least another couple of days to monitor her progress, which seems to go in fits and starts.

"She has made some forward movement," he says, "but she still has a way to go. The CT scan I had done yesterday showed that she still has excess fluid surrounding her brain, accounting for why she continues to experience head pain. The pain will probably continue for a couple of weeks more until the clotting from her hematoma and the excess fluid around it is reabsorbed into her body."

In response to our question, he says he hopes she will not have to undergo surgery.

Despite Dr. Nanda's comments, Janna remains greatly concerned. In her eyes, her mother doesn't seem to be making much progress. She hates to see her in such pain, and she can't wait to see her mother's problem vigorously addressed and her pain gone once and for all. Although she doesn't say it explicitly, it's clear she thinks that if surgery will do the trick, then bring it on.

Janna's concerns mirror similar concerns I heard for many weeks after from various friends and relatives. They never exactly came right out and said it, but their comments implied that they thought surgery to address her subdural hematoma should have been performed immediately after her accident. I, on the other hand, believed (and still do) that the more conservative approach in anything medical is the preferred one. I am keenly aware that any surgery, especially brain surgery, can carry with it unintended negative consequences. I was willing to let the neurosurgeons follow her closely, take multiple CT scans to monitor the extent of the bleeding in her skull (while recognizing that multiple doses of radiation to her head carried with it their own danger), all while participating as much as I could in her treatment planning. In other words, like the medical people, I preferred to take the more measured course dealing with this monster, while staying at the ready to raise an objection if I felt they might be going in a wrong direction.

Aware of all the potential problems that might arise in the course of, or after, surgery (and especially on such a delicate and major organ of the body), I am just as happy that neurosurgery, although a definite option, is not yet being actively planned. Joanie seems to me to be improving, although slowly and inconsistently, as the days shush-click along. At times over the previous two days she could complete a sentence, at times she had trouble finding words to complete one. At times she complained of considerable head pain, at times the pain seemed to be moderating. At times she was confused as to where she was and why, at times she was aware. This jumble of high and low notes, the neurosurgeons and her nurses keep assuring us, is to be expected with someone who has sustained a pretty hard blow to the head.

I take heart from the fact that when Joan is awake she seems to recognize Janna and me and converse a little with us and the nurses. She certainly doesn't have much "spunk," but at least she is talking. That is an improvement over her condition just two days before, when she could neither speak nor move nor tell us our daughter's name. Her face brightens momentarily when I describe the many e-mails, cards, and other expressions of concern we have gotten from relatives and friends. And she keeps repeating her mantra: "Of all the stupid things to have happen to me."

The ins and outs of lucidity Joanie demonstrated over the prior few days would become salient weeks later when she tells me that she had no recall at all of what went on for the ten-day period beginning on Friday, December 8, when, home from her first hospitalization, severe pain and nausea were sweeping over her. When I recount to her the circumstances that led to her being taken out of our house in an ambulance, she exclaims, "There were strange men in our bedroom?! What was I wearing?"

Driving home together in my car this evening, Janna says, "Pop, you know how Mom always loves to decorate the house for Christmas and put up ornaments and wreaths all over the place and decorate a tree. Let's buy a tree and decorate the house ourselves so that when she comes home, it'll feel like Christmas to her." I look over at her, but instead of seeing my grown daughter, I see her as she was as a child: thick sandy hair, impish smile, beautiful blue-green eyes. My little sweetie always reveled in hatching surprises, like the time when, as a twelve-year-old, she and a friend opened a "restaurant" in our house during one of their play dates—complete with a hand-written menu—and cooked dinner for Joanie and me. Here she is cooking up another surprise for her mother, and I have to smile to myself.

"We won't do everything she normally would do for Christmas," Janna goes on, realistically assessing that we don't have the time, what with spending every day at the hospital, "but we'll at least get the house looking like Christmas."

To Joanie, a house with all the traditional trappings of Christmas has always evoked in her warm memories of her childhood. Growing up in a small, semi-rural town southwest of Boston in a family of four, she loves Christmastime and all its small-town, Norman Rockwell traditions. She insisted, especially after our children came along, on decorating our house for the holidays. Coming from a far different background, I couldn't see what all the fuss was about, but I could see how Joanie and our children immersed themselves in, and enjoyed, it every year.

I agree with Janna that it would help Joanie's recovery if she were to come home to a house that "looked like Christmas." We decide to keep it a secret from her, and we hatch our plans.

When we arrive home, there is an e-mail from Todd waiting for us:

> *Hey, guys.*
>
> *So I thought I'd try to make it out there to Boston and spend Christmas with you guys and cheer mom up a bit. Does it matter to you when I travel? Right now there are still reasonable tickets if I leave here on 12/24 and return on 12/29 or 12/30. Although there are only a few tickets remaining, so I gotta book fast. Does that sound like a good time to travel? Should I try to get there earlier? Let me know.*
>
> *--T*

I call Todd to let him know that any of the dates he is planning to travel on are fine and that his mother might possibly be out of the hospital by then and overjoyed to see him.

I have two more things to do before going to bed. First, I compose and send an e-mail update:

> *Although she still has a way to go, Joanie is making progress. Her sodium level is normal and her*

neurological signs are good, although she still has some swelling in her brain. She still has head pain (although not as bad as previously) which, we are told, will continue for a couple of weeks more until the clotting from her hematoma gets reabsorbed into her body. Today she conversed pretty well with Janna, me, and the nurses. Her face lit up when I told her how many e-mails, cards, and other expressions of concern she has gotten from her relatives and friends . . . .

She will be moved out of the intensive care unit tomorrow (Thursday) to a regular hospital room at Lahey, and we are told that if all goes well there, she will be discharged a few days after that. Considering that she was unable to speak or move just two days ago, I am very pleased with her progress.

Second, I write a letter to Dr. Halporn to thank him for all he has done for us over and above what reasonably might be expected of a physician who had her in his care only briefly. I inform him of what I call Joan's "remarkable progress." I write further that I had met very few true altruists in my life, but that he is indeed one. I put it in our mailbox for the postal carrier to pick up tomorrow morning.

Thursday, December 14

So much for remarkable progress. When I get to the hospital, Joanie seems to be in severe pain. She sleeps less serenely than before. Instead of staying in one position, as she has done previously when napping in her hospital bed, she moves her arms alternately over her eyes in a strange, stereotyped fashion as she sleeps. It looks every bit as if she is fending off attacking demons.

Shush-click. Shush-click. Shush-click. Shush-click.

Dr. Nanda visits Joanie in the afternoon and then meets with Janna and me outside her room.

"The accumulation of fluid around her brain has increased. Let me show you her most recent CT scans," he says as he calls up her scans on the computer screen in the alcove outside her room. As he clicks on progressively more recent scans, he continues, "These show how the cerebral fluid has built up progressively and is pressing on her brain, causing its midline to move several millimeters off to one side." We peer carefully at the screen to see the midline shift he is talking about clearly demonstrated in the CT images. Then, "She's going to need surgery to drain the fluid, which I've scheduled for seven thirty tomorrow morning."

I ask Dr. Nanda for further details about the neurosurgery and what the downsides of it might be. He explains to Janna and me that once she is in the operating room, "I will make a small incision in her skin at the point on her left temple where the CT scan indicates the hematoma is located. Cutting and then parting the skin over her skull, I will next drill a small dime- or quarter-size hole, which is called a burr hole, through the exposed skull bone and drain off the blood and other fluid lying beneath it that is the product of her hematoma. This will relieve the pressure on her brain and allow it to assume its more normal symmetrical position within her skull. I will then suture the incision. All this will take about two hours.

"Once the burr hole is made, however, and I can see the actual conditions that confront us at the hematoma site, if I find that the hematoma has clotted and solidified to such an extent that it would be difficult to drain the fluid, I would have to perform a craniotomy. I know that sounds drastic, but it's really a straightforward procedure in which I extend the incision and then remove a rectangular piece of her skull to get at the clotted material. Once that material is taken out, the skull piece would be reattached and the incision sutured up. It's really not an unusual procedure," he reassures us, "but it will take about twice as long as the burr hole procedure would take."

Dr. Nanda lays out the potential downsides of the surgery. Something could go wrong, as with any neurosurgery (although because he is not intending to cut into Joanie's brain itself, but only the outer lining, there is less chance of a catastrophic misstep). And, as with any surgery, there is always a chance of infection finding its way into her body. The neurosurgeon also tells us that, even after draining the excess fluid from around her brain with this operation, he might later have to go in again should the fluid start to accumulate again.

We discuss thoroughly with him the upsides and downsides of the procedure as we understand it. I am pretty frightened at this point for Joanie, for although Dr. Nanda minimized the severity of a craniotomy, it sounds pretty drastic to me. Janna, so glad that her mother's problems and pain are now going to be addressed aggressively, expresses her opinion clearly to the neurosurgeon: "Do what you have to do to finally make her better." Seeing her mother in so much pain, Janna is all too ready to have the surgery proceed. At this point, so am I.

We go back into Joanie's room while Dr. Nanda tells her she needs an operation to remove the excess fluid that has accumulated and explains briefly what he is planning to do. Joanie's head pain is so severe that she can barely respond to him, but when she hears that the operation likely will relieve it, she gives her assent for it readily. A nurse gives us a number of papers to review and sign that will allow the surgery to proceed. We discuss them with Joanie, but it is apparent that she is in no condition to process all the information or to make any further decisions. As her health care proxy, I sign the papers.

Janna and I stay with Joanie while she alternately naps and asks us a few questions about the surgery. We try to break it gently to her that the surgery team will be drilling into her skull to get at the accumulating fluid, and that they might possibly even have to remove a larger piece of her skull to get at it. We tell her that if the latter is the case, the bone will be put back into place at the end of the operation. We assure her that after the operation, her head pain will decrease. Her response to all this information is subdued—whether from the enormity of it all or just because she is unable to process it is unclear. She mostly just stares at us.

Shush-click. Shush-click. Shush-click. Shush-click.

When the evening shift comes on at seven o'clock, we leave for home so that the three of us can get a decent night's rest before the surgery tomorrow morning.

On the way home, I call Todd from my cell phone to fill him in on this latest development and on what is being planned and to answer his questions as best I can about his mother's rapidly changing condition and the planned neurosurgery.

"I'm moving my trip up, Dad," he tells me. "I'm going to fly in as early as I can get reservations for." I agree that it will do his mother a world of good at this point to see him and then ring off so he can rearrange his flight reservations.

Several months later, Todd tells me, "I think just from my point of view of the whole incident, it seemed like I hadn't gotten an idea of how serious Mom's situation was until she actually had surgery . . . . My impression of the incident before then was that she just had the equivalent of a mild concussion and was going to be okay. I think this is a combination of your trying not to worry me about the situation and putting a bit of a positive spin on things (so that it wouldn't seem too upsetting), and the fact that I remember talking to her the day she got back from Emerson the first time, and she seemed fine. So it was kind of a surprise to me that things got as bad as they did."

Shortly after we arrive home, tired and anxious, I receive a phone call from an anesthesiology resident at Lahey, who discusses with me the four medications they are planning to give Joanie for the surgery tomorrow morning. She wants me to understand completely the risks and benefits of the drugs they will be giving her. She answers my questions about them and their effects. Janna and I make something to eat, wash up, and prepare for bed.

At quarter to ten, as we are each preparing to go to our rooms to sleep, I receive another phone call, this time from Dr. Nanda's resident, Dr. Hoit.

"Your wife's blood sodium level has dropped, and the swelling in her cranium has increased, endangering her. We're not going to wait until tomorrow morning to perform the surgery. We're going to operate on her at eleven o'clock tonight."

I tell Janna about the phone call, and she and I hurriedly change back into our clothes—jeans and a shirt for each of us—and leave for the hospital. Fortunately, traffic at this hour is very light, and we make it to Joanie's room in the SICU by ten thirty. This gives us an opportunity to spend some time with her before the operation, but she is not very aware of our presence.

At quarter to eleven, Dr. Nanda, dressed in short-sleeve surgical blues, along with the anesthesiologist and two surgical nurses, all similarly attired, come in to wheel Joanie into the operating room. He tells us that he will come to the SICU waiting room as soon as the surgery is over to tell us how it went and to discuss Joanie's condition with us. His team then wheels her bed through the doors heading toward the surgery suite.

As they do, I choke up but manage to blurt out to them, "Take good care of my girl."

Janna and I go into the Surgical Intensive Care Unit's waiting room to await Dr. Nanda's report of the surgery's outcome, glad that Lahey Clinic has thought enough about the comfort of patients' families to provide reclining chairs for waiting family members to rest in. I am also glad that neither the Queen of the Waiting Room, nor anyone else for that matter, is there, for both Janna and I each have a lot to sort through. Although my head is spinning from the rapid march of events and thoughts of what might go wrong, I am comforted by Dr. Nanda's confidence in his ability, his forthrightness in explaining his surgical plan to us, and the generally good feeling I have about this hospital and this neurosurgeon. With fatigue overtaking me, I even manage to get in a couple of catnaps during our wait for the results of the surgery. Janna, who's never acquired my ability to take short naps, stays awake the whole time.

Friday, December 15

I awake with a start at one o'clock, exactly two hours after Joanie entered the surgical suite. Dr. Nanda comes into the SICU waiting room at 1:05 a.m. The room is still quiet and devoid of people, save Janna and me.

"The surgery went well. I only had to do the burr hole procedure," he reports. "We drained off a considerable amount of fluid from around her brain; we left a tube in her scalp near the site of the surgery to drain any further fluid that might accumulate there. I'm planning to leave it in for a couple of days. The breathing tube that we inserted into her to help her breathe during the operation is even out; shortly after the surgery was over, she was able to breathe on her own."

At this point, both Janna and I breathe a lot easier ourselves.

We visit Joanie for a while back in her room. She is groggy and hardly awake, but she seems to recognize us and to be in less pain. Janna glares at Joanie's head and then gives me a sidelong glance. Unspoken between us is the fact that we were both expecting to see a small incision and a few stitches on her temple for the burr hole, but instead, we are shocked to see that the hair on the entire left side of her head has been shaved, and there is a nine-inch-long incision there. The incision follows her hairline in an arc from the center of her forehead, up around her hairline, and down to her left temple.

This larger incision was made, I was told later, in order to fold her skin down to get at the burr hole site without leaving a visible scar on her forehead, but right now, it is upsetting to both Janna and me to see the unexpectedly large cut that's been made in the skin on her head. Her left eye—on the side where they had pulled down the skin flap to get at the spot on her exposed skull at which to drill the burr hole—is bruised and swollen. She has about thirty brownish-red stitches along the incision, all of which is covered loosely with a dressing. The stitches along the curve of the incision look to me like nothing other than the stitching on a baseball.

A drain tube from under her scalp, a few inches rearward of the midpoint of the incision, is connected to a receptacle that rests behind her on the pillow. Any additional fluid that might collect around her brain will be drained off into this receptacle. Lying there with her head shaved, all those stitches looking like a seamstress's practice, the dressing on top, the drain tube coming out of her head, the swelling and bruising around her eye, all I can think is that, at this moment, Joanie looks beautiful to me.

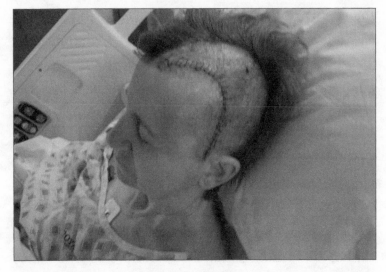

Baseball stitching.

Shush-click. Shush-click. Shush-click. Shush-click.

The nurse kicks us out after a short while, telling us to go home and get some sleep. "You look like you could use some," she adds.

Ω Ω Ω

I wake up at home late in the morning, not exactly refreshed, but much relieved. Janna is still sleeping. In the morning's quiet, I send an e-mail to update everyone about the latest developments:

> *As Joanie's hematoma dissolved, it produced a lot of fluid that was exerting pressure on her brain and causing her considerable pain. Consequently, she had a surgical procedure done last night to drain the*

excess fluid. The neurosurgeon made an incision in her scalp and then drilled a dime-sized burr hole through her skull to drain off the blood. He told us that they drained a lot of blood and fluid off (easing the pressure on her brain), and that after the procedure was finished Joanie could respond to commands and didn't need a breathing tube (i.e., could breathe on her own). Janna and I were with Joanie both before they took her to the OR (10:45 p.m.) and afterward in her room in the Intensive Care Unit right after the operation (1:00 a.m.). She was groggy afterward but seemed to recognize us and to be in less pain. They kicked us out around 2:00 a.m.—understandably, Joanie needs rest.

The neurosurgeon who has been following Joanie since she was admitted to Lahey Clinic (a very competent and nice man) will of course continue to follow her in the ICU to take further CT scans of her head, see how much fluid continues to accumulate, check her sodium levels and neurological signs, etc. It is possible that they may have to go in again and drain off fluid again at some point. Only time will tell.

Janna and I are going to take it easy this morning, and then we'll be going in to see Joanie.

I call Todd, reaching him in California before he leaves for work, to tell him the good news that his mother's neurosurgery went well. He, in turn, gives me the good news that he was able to get a flight in to

Boston for December 20. We will all be together again in just five days.

I leave to do some errands, get a haircut I had been putting off getting, and then go to the hospital to be with Joanie. Joanie has been my barber (for what little hair I have left) for the last ten years. With her being out of commission now, I have to have my hair cut at a regular barber shop this time, which I don't like. Janna comes to the hospital later in the day in her own car, and we stay with Joan, who is awake but subdued most of the time, until the shift change at seven o'clock. Joanie is obviously tired from all that she has been through since last evening and doesn't say much to us.

After we leave her room in the SICU, Janna and I exclaim, almost simultaneously, "Whew, I'm glad the surgery was pushed up." Having it sprung on us was, all things considered, a boon—for Joanie because it relieved her pain eight hours sooner, and for the rest of the family because it averted an additional eight hours of anxiety and concern we would have gone through had we had to wait and worry about her neurosurgery for another night.

Saturday, December 16

Awake and in less pain than previously, Joanie is still slow in thought and speech, continues to perseverate, and shows both short- and long-term memory gaps.

"Was I operated on?" she asks Janna and me several times as she reaches up absently to the dressing covering her sutured incision and tries to brush it off.

As might be expected for someone who has just had a major operation, she remains subdued. We stay the day just watching her as the nurses come in and out to tend to her, observe her, and record her vital signs.

Shush-click. Shush-click. Shush-click. Shush-click.

I continue to worry about whether the aphasia I am seeing will become permanent, and thus far my attempts to find out from the physicians what they think about this have been unsuccessful. For one thing, they really can't predict her outcome (or anyone else's in a similar situation). But for another, I get the feeling that, as surgeons, they are focused primarily on her surgical healing and only secondarily on her cognitive outcome. I want to alert them to the fact that her thought and speech are not up to the level I normally see in her. Joanie is a very intelligent person, and her cognitive functioning now, while it might appear minimally "okay" to someone who does not know her well, is, to someone who does, certainly not as crisp and lucid as it was before the accident.

I know that Dr. Nanda is off duty for the weekend, but I hope at least to speak with one of his associates about my concerns. I ask the nurse on duty to relay a message about those concerns to someone in Dr. Nanda's group.

Sunday, December 17

In response to the message I left with the nurse, I receive an early morning phone call at home from Dr. Jeffrey Arle, the neurosurgeon covering for Dr. Nanda for the weekend. In a twenty-minute-long conversation, I express my concerns about Joan's apparent cognitive impairment. Dr. Arle speaks at length about all the possible impacts on cognitive functioning of the kind of injury and the kind of neurosurgery that Joan has gone through.

"There's no way to tell at this point what the specific impacts on her might be and if and when they might emerge," he says. I really don't expect him to be able to predict the future about this. My main objective in speaking with him is to register my concern about Joanie's current ability to recognize and remember things and to get the neurosurgical team to look beyond her physical healing process and attend to her cognitive healing.

On our visit to the hospital later in the morning, Janna and I find Joan to be sometimes lucid and clear, sometimes foggy. We take our cues from Joan in deciding whether or not to try to talk with her. Mostly, we don't, and she dozes on and off. While we are there, a physician assistant comes in to remove the drain from her head and to stitch the incision that had been made to accommodate it. Little fluid has drained off in the two days since her surgery (a good sign), and there is a fear that if the drain tube were to remain there longer, infection might find its way through the opening in her skin.

With the operation behind us, and Christmas only a week away, this evening Janna and I revisit her idea of readying the house for the holiday and, we hope, Joanie's homecoming. Our daughter spends half an hour in our attic going through all the boxes of decorations stored there. Over the years, as our collection of ornaments and decorations grew, Joanie characteristically organized and labeled everything down to the finest detail, so it doesn't take long for Janna to find the boxes she needs for the decorations she wants to put up and to bring them downstairs.

Before going to sleep, Janna and I (but it is mostly Janna) set about starting to make the house look like Christmas. She scurries to position around the house the brass horn, garlands, Christmas stockings, and miniature hand-crafted evergreen trees, Santa Clauses, and elves that Joanie has accumulated over the years. By the time she is finished, it still isn't half of what Joanie would normally have placed over the course of several days' decorating before the holiday, but it achieves its purpose: the house "looks like Christmas."

Monday, December 18

Joanie eats well this morning. She remains quite forgetful, however, bringing up a topic in conversation or asking a question that we had talked about only a half-hour or so before. Each time, Janna or I patiently repeat what we had said before and silently hope that this forgetfulness and perseveration will disappear with time.

Dr. Hoit comes in to check on Joanie and tells us that she is doing well. I seize the opportunity to ask him what plans are being made to deal with her memory and speech problems.

"Once she's out of intensive care and on a regular hospital floor, she'll be seen by an occupational therapist and a physical therapist. After being released from the hospital, she could have rehabilitation, either at a rehabilitation facility or at home," he replies.

This is news to us, but very welcome news, for at last I am hearing that some consideration is being given to other aspects of her recovery than solely her surgical recovery.

Dr. Hoit reveals another piece of good news: Joanie will be transferred out of the Surgical Intensive Care Unit later this evening to what the hospital calls a "Step Down" unit. He explains that this is a unit halfway in intensity of care between an intensive care unit and a regular hospital floor. The various lines and leads that were inserted into, or placed on, her will remain so they can maintain the continuous monitoring of her vital signs, but she will be given the opportunity to do a bit more than just lie in bed. Later this evening, she is moved to 6 West, the Step Down floor. Janna and I spend some time with her in her "new digs"—a large private room—where Joanie is now more animated and clearly happier. I am amazed at her body's capacity to recoup its vitality after so serious an operation has been performed on her less than four days before.

Janna and I leave for home, elated about the concrete signs of progress we are seeing. After we leave, Joanie is taken down for what will be the final CT scan of her stay at the Lahey Clinic hospital.

Tuesday, December 19

A physical therapist and an occupational therapist come to see Joanie bright and early. They disconnect various lines tethering her to her monitoring apparatus. With these removed, Joan is free to stand and to walk, which she does as the two young women observe and evaluate her movement, coordination, strength, and balance. She is encouraged to spend some time sitting in a chair in order to get the various parts of her body in positions different from when she was lying down. They comment that her motor functioning appears to be good (a testament to the fact that Joanie kept herself in good condition before her accident through exercise and good nutrition).

I express to the two therapists my considerable satisfaction about her physical condition but feel I need to keep harping about her cognitive condition. I comment that, while her motor functioning appears good, her speech and thought are still cloudy and slow. I ask them what is going to be done about that. They reply that Joanie will be further evaluated before discharge and a rehabilitation plan made for her. Finally, I am beginning to hear about possible cognitive rehabilitation.

Equipped with a walker that the therapists had brought with them, Joanie gets out of bed to navigate around the room. It is then she sees herself in a mirror for the first time since she was admitted to the hospital. She gasps. The extent to which her head was shaved and the length of the incision come as a surprise to her, just as it had to Janna and me when we first saw it. Joanie has been thinking all along that she has just a small incision somewhere along her scalp line; she had no idea that it arcs along half the length of her hairline.

"Of all the stupid things . . ." she mutters once more as she gazes at herself in the mirror.

That aside, Joanie takes joy in being free to move about, however slowly and carefully it has to be. She sits up in a chair for four hours today, tolerating it well, considering that she's been flat in bed for most of the previous eight days. She still has some head pain, and she still is not as active or awake as she normally would be during the day, but all in all, things appear to be going well for her physically.

Another sign of progress: after less than twenty-four hours in the Step Down unit, she is moved to a regular hospital room on 7 Central—the final stop before going home. We are told that if her blood sodium level, which has been good recently, remains stabilized, and if the recent CT scan does not show any signs of fluid accumulation, she will be discharged from the hospital in a day or two.

In preparation for that, the intravenous port that had been in her arm for the last eight days is removed. Her left wrist is swollen from having it there for so long, but she considers that a small price to pay for being finally free of it.

The evening's e-mail update starts with the news that Joanie has been moved from SICU to the "step-down" unit, and then from there to a regular hospital room.

> *The next step up from that is out of the hospital (either to home or to a rehab facility). They are saying that it is possible she may be discharged this week, but that all depends on how well she continues to progress. Joanie still has some head pain and is still not as active or awake as she normally would be during the day, but each day sees some improvement.*
>
> *The other day, we brought in all the get well cards and well-wishes that people have sent and read them to her. She was so pleased to hear them all. Since Janna and I have been spending most of our waking hours at the hospital with Joan, I'm sure you understand that I cannot respond individually to your*

e-mails and messages but I want to let you know, in
this collective and somewhat impersonal way, that we
all (especially Joanie) appreciate your get well wishes
and expressions of support.

Todd will be coming in from California in a
couple of days and will stay through the end of the
month. That will also undoubtedly cheer Joanie
even more, as it will mean that the four of us will be
together over the holidays.

Wednesday, December 20

With her discharge imminent, I need to buy a tree if
we are going to complete decorating the house for
Christmas by the time Joanie comes back home. I spend
the morning shopping for one. It can't be just any old
tree, though. Joanie always insisted on getting "a Fraser
fir, as fresh as it could be," which meant going to a tree
farm to cut one ourselves. There is no time to do that
now, so I go to several places to examine and then shake
their already-cut trees to get "a Fraser fir, as fresh as it
could be" for Joanie's homecoming.

Janna and I agreed last night that while I was doing
that, she would go in to visit Joanie this morning and
then leave in the afternoon (rather than at night, as
she usually did). Not only does she have to go back to
her apartment, for the first time in a week, to get clean
clothes to wear and to retrieve her mail, but also she
is to pick Todd up at Logan Airport at eleven o'clock

tonight. Since her apartment is just outside of Boston, we had agreed that she would be the one to drive in to the airport to get him.

We have not yet told Joanie that Todd moved up his planned arrival from December 24 by four days, as we thought it best for her to regain as much of her physical and cognitive functioning as possible in order to better handle the excitement of his coming in. Once I arrive at Joanie's room, shortly before noon, Janna and I tell her the news. The broad smile and glow that light up her face tells us she couldn't be happier. This afternoon, she sits in a chair for several hours, orders up by telephone her food from the hospital food service, eats well, walks around the halls, and allows herself to think that she might actually be discharged from the hospital and home in time for Christmas— and with her whole family around her.

We are soon visited by Denise Habarta, a nurse who introduces herself as Joanie's case manager. She proceeds to describe the various rehabilitation therapies available to Joan upon her discharge and asks us if we want to avail ourselves of those services at home or in a rehabilitation facility. It doesn't take Janna, Joan, and me much time to agree that home would be the best place for her. Ms. Habarta indicates that, shortly after her discharge from the hospital, a visiting nurse will come to our home, and that a physical therapist, occupational therapist, and speech therapist will be arranged for Joanie.

Then she asks if the nursing and medical staff have left any of our questions unanswered at this point. I answer forcefully that there is one: "What is the state of Joanie's cognitive functioning, and, more to the point, what specifically is going to be done to get it back to its pre-injury level?" Ms. Habarta leaves saying that she will contact Dr. Nanda and make sure that someone addresses our concerns with specific details of a rehabilitation plan.

On arriving home from the hospital, I have one more thing to do before going to bed. I put the lights up on the Christmas tree and (knowing that Todd and Janna will finish decorating it once they arrive home from the airport) place upon it just a few of the ornaments Janna had brought down from the attic. As I place each of the ornaments we had given annually to our children in earlier Christmases—like the little soccer player enthusiastically kicking a ball and the ornament with the slate on it saying "For the best teacher" we had given to Janna in years past, and the miniature computer and Yale bulldog ornaments we had given to Todd—I think back to those Christmases past when we were all together. And I look forward to this Christmas present, when we will all be home together again.

Thursday, December 21
Janna goes to the hospital early to wash and dress her mother in preparation for Todd's first visit. I drive in later with Todd, giving him the chance to sleep in after

having arrived from the airport late last night. When we arrive at her room, Joanie lights up on seeing her good-looking, blue-eyed son, and Janna and I look on at a very happy mother and son reunion. Todd looks immensely relieved to be seeing his mother finally, rather than having to hear about her from Janna or me at a distance of 3,000 miles. Joanie hugs Todd joyously.

"Bring me up to date on how you feel now, Mom," Todd requests, and pretty soon they fall into casual conversation about her hospital stay and operation and about what is new in his and Brooke's lives. Todd has a way of picking up where he had left off in his last conversation with us, and we soon all dive into a torrent of conversation.

As we chat, a nurse comes in and tells us that Joan will be discharged from the hospital today pending Dr. Nanda's review of her case and her latest CT scan to make sure that her progress has remained satisfactory.

Ms. Habarta was true to her word to have Dr. Nanda's neurosurgical team address my concerns about what would be done to try to bring Joan's speech and thought back to her pre-injury levels. We receive a visit from a nurse practitioner, David Melzack, an integral member of Dr. Nanda's neurosurgical team, and from what he says, it is clear that Ms. Habarta had gotten the team's attention about my concerns.

"Given the traumatic brain injury she suffered," Mr. Melzack tells us, "it will take time for Joan to get back to her previous level of cognitive functioning, but with time and the planned rehabilitation therapy that I'll detail for you in a minute, our neurosurgical team is confident that she will." On hearing the concrete plans he then spells out for us and his specific comments about her prognosis, our family's sigh of relief is almost audible.

A short time later, Dr. Nanda comes in to give us the good news himself that Joanie is free to leave the hospital once the discharge papers are prepared and reviewed with us. Smiles break out on all our faces: we are so happy finally to be receiving this news. He asks if we have any questions, and I tell him that I have just one that had been nagging at both Janna and me since Joan's surgery was done. "Why was the incision you made for the burr hole so extensive when it was my understanding that the procedure required only a small incision on her temple?"

Dr. Nanda explains that the imaging of her head revealed that the best place for the burr hole was on her temple, about an inch above her left eyebrow, and if he made the incision there, it would have left a visible scar. He opted, instead, to make the longer, arcing incision just inside her hairline so that once her hair grew back, the scar would not be visible. That incision required him to pull her skin down to get to the burr hole site, but it saved her from having a noticeable scar on her temple. It also explains why there had been so much bruising around her eye after the operation. He reminds me that he had quickly discussed this with me in his early morning debriefing after Joanie's surgery, but in my state of anxiety or sleepiness then (I suspect both), it hadn't sunk in.

I also later satisfy my curiosity, by doing a little research on my own, as to what kind of instrument was used to drill that hole in her skull. It was indeed a kind of drill, called a "perforator." This instrument has a carefully designed and precision-built tip that allows the surgeon to apply firm and consistent pressure on the skull bone but stops the cutting action as soon as it goes through it, "thereby protecting all that is soft underneath," Katrina Firlik, a neurosurgeon has written. She goes on: "What you are left with is a nice, smooth, round, full-thickness hole in the skull, roughly nickel-size in diameter. Believe me, this was a great breakthrough in the history of neurosurgery." Believe *me* when I say thank goodness for this neurosurgical invention.

At one thirty in the afternoon, the nurse arrives with Joanie's discharge papers, instructions on her care and the medications she should take while recovering, and a list of the therapists who will be contacting us for follow-up rehabilitation at home. She admonishes Joanie that she will have to take it easy for quite a while to give all her bodily systems a chance to recover and reintegrate, but she assures us that recovery will come with time. With that, we wait for a wheelchair to come to take Joanie from her room and out of the hospital.

As we wait, I gaze over at my wife. Her head is bald where they had shaved her to get to the hematoma that had assaulted her brain, she still is sporting thirty stitches from the surgery, and she is pale and weak from having been in bed for so long, but she looks as good and happy as I had seen her look at any time over the past three weeks.

Soon, the wheelchair arrives to take her down to the hospital entrance. The worst thing that can happen to someone with a traumatic brain injury is to hit her head again within a year of the original injury, and I think to myself how terrible it would be if we were to get in a traffic accident while we are driving home. So when I pull my car up to the hospital entrance, we place Joanie—like a fragile egg—in the safest part of the car, the middle of the rear seat. Todd gets in beside her, and Janna goes to get her car from the parking garage. By prior arrangement, I am to drive home slowly to allow Janna time to get home before me so she can turn on the lights of the Christmas trees, the little artificial one in the breezeway and the large, real one in the family room. I would have driven home slowly anyway, given the delicate cargo I am carrying.

As we pass the Burlington Mall on the drive home, I point it out to Joanie. I want to make concrete the answers Janna and I had given to the question she asked us so many times while in the hospital, the one about just where the Lahey Clinic is located. Halfway home, she remarks, "How terrible it must have been for you and Janna to have to drive all this way to get to the hospital to visit me." In actuality, it is only a thirty-minute drive, but to Joanie, the drive home must seem as if it were taking forever.

She also comments how strange everything looks. Over and above having been groggy and confused so much over the past several weeks, she also has been in an environment that was sensorily restricted. All that she had seen during that time were the confines of a room, either a hospital room or, when she was home between hospitalizations, our bedroom. Now she is emerging into the light, so to speak, and certainly into surroundings that are infinitely busier, with sights and sounds she's not seen for weeks.

When we arrive home, Todd and I gingerly help Joanie out of the car. On entering our breezeway, she notices the little artificial Christmas tree we had decorated and placed there and says, "Oh, you got the little tree down. That's nice."

Then she walks into the house and sees the decorations Janna had put up all over the house and the Christmas tree we had bought and trimmed, its lights ablaze. She bursts into tears. She sits on the family room sofa, her eyes darting from place to place around the family room, like a frightened animal in a new environment, taking in the live Christmas tree Janna and Todd had decorated and all the other decorations there. Recovering her composure, she says, "This is so wonderful, just being here together in our own house."

She is home at last, and, yes, the four of us are together again, and, yes, it is wonderful being all together and back home. Now begins the work of getting Joanie back to normal.

6

REHABILITATION

Friday, December 22

WITH JOANIE BACK HOME now, we are still unsure what her recovery will entail. We have the outline of a rehabilitation plan but are unclear about how that will play itself out. Having been on her back in bed for most of the three preceding weeks, what muscular strength and coordination has she lost during that time? Will she return to the level of physical ability she had before her injury, and how soon? And the question that burns most intensely in our minds: would she regain the mental abilities she has lost? It doesn't take long before we begin down the road that will give us answers to these questions.

The phone rings shortly after nine a.m. It is Christine Thomasch, a visiting nurse from Emerson Hospital Home Care, a part of Emerson Hospital that provides home-based rehabilitation. She is calling to say she would like to see Joanie today. We arrange a time and then, shortly afterward, Laurie Thibodeau, an occupational therapist from the same organization, calls to arrange a visit for today, too. I hope these rehabilitation people are as good as they are fast.

The nurse arrives a little later in her SUV, toting a bag containing various items of equipment of her profession, including a laptop computer. Beginning a practice we will engage in whenever Joanie has a home-based rehabilitation session, whoever else is at home will sit on the tan leather love seat in our family room and observe what goes on and how Joanie reacts. Because we also may be called in to help her later in the activities and exercises she's given to help improve her functioning, we feel we should be in on these sessions. Joanie doesn't mind our presence at these times. In fact, she gives every indication of wanting us there to add support and bolster her confidence, learn more about her condition as the rehabilitation specialists see it, and help her recall aspects of the session she might forget.

It is immediately clear that Ms. Thomasch is aware of the history of my wife's accident and her general medical history, but she asks Joanie a few questions just the same to put her at ease and clarify some details. She takes her vital signs, makes an on-the-spot nursing followup plan that she reviews with us and has us sign, and tells us that a different visiting nurse will be meeting with Joan during the course of her rehabilitation.

Later, Laurie Thibodeau, who will be Joan's occupational therapist for her home-based rehabilitation, arrives, also in an SUV, also toting a bag containing equipment of her profession and a laptop computer. As we are to discover in the days ahead, an SUV, equipment bag, and laptop are apparently standard kit for the Emerson Hospital Home Care therapists— whether by coincidence or design, we never fathom.

Again, Todd, Janna, and I look on as Laurie goes through the same initial ritual with Joanie as the nurse did earlier, asking her for clarifying details about her accident and subsequent hospital stays. She then does an evaluation of her physical condition, observing Joanie as she walks, testing her arm and leg strength, and noting how well she regains her balance when she pushes against her. She concludes that she has some weakness on the right side of her body and some balance problems, neither of them, in her estimation, terribly severe nor likely to be permanent. Given that Joan has spent essentially the past three weeks lying in bed, these physical impairments are not wholly unexpected nor alarming. Laurie also comments (as will the other rehabilitation therapists that come through) that Joanie appears to have kept herself in good physical condition, which augurs well for her eventual recovery to normal physical functioning.

Laurie takes a brief tour through our house in order to make recommendations about how best to cope with Joanie's temporary balance and strength issues so that she can carry out daily activities safely. As we had heard from the physicians and nurses during her hospitalization, and as Laurie reiterates, the worst thing that can happen to Joanie during the first year after her injury would be to suffer another fall that injures her head. Laurie recommends, at least until Joanie regains her strength and balance, that a member of the family follow her up and down the stairs in case she loses her balance, and that she should take showers seated on a shower seat (which we subsequently borrow from a local agency). When she is up to going outside of the house, Laurie directs her not to go unaccompanied because outside surfaces are a lot more uneven than those in a house. She also recommends one permanent change: that we install a grab bar in our shower stall.

Laurie advises us that the patient should not hurry to resume any normal activity until she feels ready to do it safely. Of course, we don't intend to let Joanie resume any normal housekeeping activities while she is recovering, even if she wants to (which, at this point, she doesn't anyway). Todd, Janna, and I figure no housework for her, no driving, perhaps not even any visits from friends until Joanie feels up to it. We make a plan for our meals over the next several days and a shopping list to go along with it.

Joanie badly wants her hair washed, as it has been a long time since its last washing. Laurie okays this for the half of her head that does not have stitches on it. After Laurie leaves, Janna gives her mother a half-shampoo as Joanie leans over the kitchen sink.

I want to be sure, now that she no longer has hospital nurses administering her medications, that there is no doubt about what medications Joanie should take and when she should take them. She has been prescribed four drugs to take at home: Keppra, a precautionary medicine to avert seizures; Fioricet for her head pain; and Senna and Colace, a laxative and stool softener, respectively, to counteract the constipation often caused by the pain medication. Some of these are to be taken twice a day, some once, and some only when and if needed. I want to be absolutely certain that there will be no confusion about any of this—that if I give her her morning medications, she will not, given her cognitive state, inadvertently repeat them, nor would Janna or Todd unknowingly give her a repeat dose. Consequently, I list the various medications she is to take and the instructions for taking them on the left side of a sheet of paper, write dates across the top, and give strict instructions to everyone in the house to record the time, under the proper date, when Joan takes each pill.

There is much to tell our friends and relatives about the past three days, but little time to do it. I hurriedly compose an e-mail update to tell everyone that our patient is home.

Joanie was discharged from the hospital yesterday (Thursday) and is now home. She has to take it easy while all her systems have a chance to recover. Over the next couple of months, she'll have all kinds of therapists (physical, occupational, speech) coming to the house to help that process along. Today, already, she's had visits from a nurse and the occupational therapist. Next week she has the stitches from her incision removed, and the week after that she'll have a CT scan to check on whether or not any more fluid is accumulating around her brain, and the week after that she'll have an appointment with the neurosurgeon who did the surgery.

Todd came in from California on Wednesday and will stay until just before New Year's, and Janna's school is off for the holidays, so she is staying here until after New Year's. Between the three of us and the many visiting therapists, she'll get lots of attentive recuperative care over the coming weeks. She's still not up to talking on the phone or having visitors. It will take time before she's back to her old self, but we are hoping for her full recovery. With Joanie now out of the hospital and finally home, we're going to have the best of holiday seasons. I wish you the same.

Saturday, December 23

Todd (who's a foodie and an enthusiastic cook) and I make plans to go to the supermarket in the afternoon to buy what we will need to implement our meal plan.

Before we can, however, I receive a call from another Emerson Hospital Home Care worker, Ursula Horst, a physical therapist. She wants to evaluate the patient later today and make a plan for her physical rehabilitation.

When another SUV pulls into our driveway, we know it has to be she. Like the others, she asks Joanie some questions about her fall, her operation, and her hospitalizations. Then she asks, "And so how are you feeling now?"

It takes Joanie only a second to answer: "Well, kind of royally pissed off that the whole thing happened, I guess." Sympathetic nods all around as we muffle our giggles.

Ursula's evaluation of Joan's physical condition consists of asking her questions about her accident and what changes it has wrought to her physically, watching her walk, having her pull the therapist's arm while the therapist resists her efforts, asking Joan to stand while she sees how much force it takes to throw her off balance, and similar tests of strength, coordination, and balance. After her evaluation, Ursula devises a plan for Joan's physical therapy that focuses on returning her core strength to its pre-accident level, working on her balance, and generally getting her large muscle strength back to where it was before. Another physical therapist, Tricia Reed, will come in once or twice a week, Ursula tells us, to provide exercises to help the patient achieve these objectives. As she improves over the next few weeks, she goes on, Joanie might want to begin to do rehabilitative exercises in an outpatient facility that has specific equipment for it. Like the other rehabilitation visitors, she remarks how basically good Joan's physical prowess is considering how severe her initial injury was. Ursula says that she expects her to make good progress over the next few weeks toward returning to her pre-accident level of physical functioning. All the rehab people are very encouraging throughout the rehabilitation period.

As her mind begins to clear from her hospitalizations, Joanie starts to express the desire to get back to her normal activities, especially to get back to walking to the Bean. These daily three-mile round trips to Boston Bean House truly had been her "zen moment" every day, and she can't wait to resume these walks. She has used them to clear her mind as well as exercise her body. Joan asks Ursula when she might be able to make the daily walks on her own, but Ursula doesn't give her a specific reply. Instead, she says that, given Joanie's good underlying physical conditioning and her adherence to the exercises she is recommending, she is confident she can resume her daily walks in the near future.

There is another reason Joanie wants to get back to Boston Bean. Aside from enjoying her power walk to the coffee shop and back, and the coffee and scones on offer there, both she and I enjoy the crowd there. In the ten years the shop has been open in the heart of

Maynard, we have become friendly with its owners and the other regular customers. Dawn and Eli Schallhorn, the owners, and the counter staff, young Eli (their son), Gabe, and Maria, have provided a homey atmosphere in the shop that has allowed customers, owners, and counter workers to coalesce into a real community, and an easy familiarity among these three groups has developed. Joanie really misses the gang at the Bean, and, as is evident from the cards and the elaborate live plant basket they sent while she was in the hospital, they miss Joanie.

After Todd and I finish our delayed shopping at the supermarket in the afternoon, he asks me to stop the car at the nearby Starbuck's.

"I'll be right back, Dad. Just wait here for me." He returns with a cup of coffee in one hand and a bag containing a scone for his mother in the other. One of Joanie's favorite treats that she occasionally allows herself to indulge in is a scone. When we get home and he gives it to her, she smiles a big smile and gives Todd a big hug.

Sunday, December 24

Maybe the film is called *Never on Sunday*, but Nancy Carolus, the visiting nurse, comes on this Sunday to check on Joanie. She asks her how she is doing, to which Joanie replies "I'm beginning to feel better, but it would be so good to be back to normal." She relates that she feels both her reading ability and her memory have suffered as a result of the accident. Nancy assures us all that Joan's reading and similar activities will frustrate her for a while, especially when she is tired, but that those capabilities will come back to pre-accident levels gradually.

I can understand Joan's frustration. Here is a woman who has earned a doctorate, managed a household, raised two children to productive adulthood, and who, before the accident, was sharp as a tack. Yet we all (including her) can't help but notice that ideas that had tripped readily off her tongue before are now clouded by hesitation. Her speech is slower and punctuated by pauses as she searches for the next words. She loves to read, solve puzzles, and play word games, yet here she is, though still able to read, impeded in that ability. When she reads something to us, such as a Christmas card, we see that some words are just a blank to her, and she has to ask for help. It breaks my heart to see her this way, but I hope (even if I don't know for certain) that she will regain these lost capacities. This is a temporary disruption, I tell myself and her, not a permanent condition. But I really don't know that for sure.

Todd, Janna, and I can see, as she watches her favorite TV word game shows—*Wheel of Fortune* and *Jeopardy*—since coming home from the hospital that she is having difficulty solving puzzles that she routinely would have solved long before the rest of us. Usually, she zips through the *New York Times* Sunday crossword puzzles with no trouble, but since she has come home, she cannot complete even one.

Seeing this, Todd calls me aside and suggests, out of his mother's earshot, that he print off some of the easier, weekday *New York Times* puzzles for her, using his on-line subscription, to give to her later when she is more up to the challenge. He points out that his wife, Brooke, who is a nurse, had recently attended a lecture on brain injury at which the lecturer advised care-givers not to stimulate patients' thinking too early, as this would do more harm than good. We agree to hold even the easy *Times* crossword puzzles aside to give to her at a later time when it appears that she is ready to attack them.

All of this trouble with speaking, thinking, and reading causes Joanie to shy away from using the telephone, working on the computer, using e-mail, and talking to people outside the family. This is typical of people who have sustained traumatic brain injuries, especially in the speech and language centers of the brain, as Joan has. For the next several weeks, virtually all of her communications to and from the world outside of our immediate family—that normally would have involved her using the telephone or e-mail or talking face-to-face—come and go through Janna, Todd, or me.

With Christmas eve upon us, a neighbor and close friend of Joanie's, Lillian Ramos, pops in unexpectedly.

On seeing Joanie, she starts to cry, and on seeing Lillian cry, Joanie does the same. They embrace, recover their composure, and then go on to talk about the injury and her hospitalization. A short time later, our neighbor Mary Schatz also pays a visit, staying about fifteen minutes. They talk about normal things, like what's been going on in the neighborhood, things that help make Joanie feel she could be returning to normal.

Both Christmas eve visits cheer Joan, for she has not seen these good friends, nor they her, for almost three weeks. But I can tell that just keeping up a conversation with them has tired her out. With tomorrow being Christmas, I make sure she gets upstairs and into bed earlier than usual this evening.

Monday, December 25

Christmas Day, and the four of us are together at home. Three weeks before, we were not sure this would even happen, for in that period our family had been tipped into a crisis like we have never before experienced.

Back before Thanksgiving, before her accident, before any of this ordeal could even be imagined, Joanie discussed with me an idea she had been considering about Christmas presents.

"Since Janna and Todd and Brooke are thinking of buying condos and will have mortgages to pay off, I don't want them to go spending a lot of money on Christmas gifts. What do you think of the idea," she then proposed, "of limiting the Christmas presents among us to just one from each person? We could draw names out of a hat to determine who would give gifts to whom."

"Given that they're now really going to have to save their pennies, it sounds like a good idea," I replied. "But you know how much the kids like gift-giving at Christmas. They'd probably be disappointed at giving and getting only one gift each."

Joan and I kicked it around some more and came up with the plan that everyone in the family would give (and receive) two gifts each—a small, stocking-stuffer type of gift and a larger one (but with an upper dollar limit).

When we had all been together at Thanksgiving, we talked it over with Todd, Brooke, and Janna. We could tell that Janna was disappointed, as it is her nature to be very generous about gift-giving. Aware of her disappointment, we discussed it some more, refined the logistics a bit, and in the end we all agreed on a plan. With that, Joanie wrote each of our names on two slips of paper, put them in a hat, and we did our gift drawing.

"Remember," she cautioned our offspring, "no going overboard with the Christmas gifts. You guys are going to have to be watching your budgets from now on."

Joan's accident has gotten in the way of Christmas shopping, though, so there aren't even two gifts apiece for anyone today. This Christmas morning we each set out under the tree what few gifts we had bought before her accident had occurred. Even with all that has happened to her, Joan is apologetic that she doesn't have presents for the people whose names she had drawn. "Todd, Janna, I guess you'll have to wait a little while for your presents. Maybe 'Santa' will send you something in January sometime." They rush to assure her that that is the last thing on their minds, and I try to lighten the mood with, "It's not a 'big haul' this year, but it'll have to do for now."

I had done my shopping early and had bought, as my smaller gift for my wife, the inveterate puzzle solver, a hand-held Sudoku game. But now, with her brain injury affecting her language and problem-solving skills, I think it best not to put it out for her for Christmas. To the meager collection of family gifts we have for one another, I put under the tree a few others that friends from out-of-town had mailed us. It is not a "big haul" by any means.

After breakfast, we open the gifts. We call Brooke, who stayed in California to be with her parents, and share some of the Christmas spirit with her over the phone.

Still in our sleepwear, we sit in the family room and talk, just the four of us, just like Christmases past. Soon, Joanie returns to wondering out loud, as she often does since getting out of the hospital, "Will I ever get back to normal?" We do our best to assure her she will but that it will take time. We kid her about what an impatient patient she is and empathize with her about how frustrating it must be for her. But I keep wondering the same thing that Joanie is wondering, and I can tell that Todd and Janna do, too.

With the four of us at home, just like old times, we have our traditional Christmas dinner, just like old times: pasta and artichokes. When our children were growing up, their mother, for several years running, put together a traditional dinner of turkey or ham with different kinds of vegetables and other trimmings, only to find that the children—picky eaters that they were then—didn't eat much of it. So one Christmas, she challenged them to compose a menu themselves of food that they would really like to have, and what Todd and Janna came up with was pasta and artichokes. Ever since, that has been our traditional Christmas dinner.

This Christmas, Todd and Janna prepare the meal, with Todd making the marinara sauce and, for him and me (the only red meat eaters in the family), Italian meatballs. Janna prepares the artichokes and the dipping sauce for them and sets the table. Joanie relaxes—reluctantly, for this is normally her prerogative, but she does relax—as she watches, with loving eyes, the rest of the family prepare our traditional holiday artichokes and pasta.

We sit at the dining room table, set festively by Janna with green and red placemats and a centerpiece of little

Santa statues, to enjoy the meal. But first we have to
engage in another family ritual. When our children were
younger, we spent Christmases together with another
family, the Hewitts, who are originally from England.
They introduced us to Christmas crackers—rolled,
decorated cardboard tubes with tabs at each end—a
custom in England that hadn't caught on much in the
U.S. at that time. When the tabs on the rolled tube are
pulled (one person pulling one end and the person next
to him or her pulling the other), the cracker makes
a loud crack, and a cheesy toy, a cheesy hat, and an
equally cheesy strip of paper containing a corny joke
or riddle pop out from the tube. Some days before this
Christmas, I had purchased Christmas crackers on my
way to visit Joanie at the hospital, and now I trot them
out so we can follow our Christmas cracker tradition.

Every Christmas day, toward the end of the day,
with the opening of the gifts finished, the dinner of
pasta and artichokes behind us, the cheesy Christmas
cracker toys scattered about on the dinner table, and
the last present tried on or played with, Joanie and I
would gaze at the Christmas tree and kiddingly tell
one another "This is the best Christmas tree we've
ever had." This year, we look at the Christmas tree I
had bought in a hurry just before she came home from
the hospital, one that has nowhere near the symmetry
and beauty of trees we had bought together in more
relaxed Christmases past, one that is nowhere near as

fresh as the trees we would cut ourselves at the tree farm in years before, and a tree that has only half the decorations it normally would have had on it. I hold her tight and say, without the usual irony in my voice, "This is the best Christmas tree we've ever had. And," with even less irony, "this is the best Christmas tree we'll *ever* have because you're home now."

Tuesday, December 26

Joanie dresses in regular clothes for the first time since her accident, for we have a special appointment to keep. She will be getting her stitches removed. The four of us pile into my car and drive back to the Lahey Clinic where the suture removal is to be done by one of Dr. Nanda's physician assistants. As we walk through the lobby of the hospital where Joanie had arrived by ambulance two weeks before, she sees the hospital in its full length and breadth for the first time. Arrayed around the large lobby are a cafeteria, a coffee shop, a gift shop, a travel agency, an optician's office, a pharmacy, a busy information desk, and other offices and shops offering support and services to patients, families, and visitors, some of whom come from far away. Someone is tinkling melodies on the grand piano in the lobby, the cafeteria is running full bore, and patients, visitors, and staff are scurrying in all directions. Joanie blinks at it all and remarks how big and bustling the hospital is and how imposing its lobby looks to her.

She is trying, in her mind, to place herself within this institution where she had just spent ten days of her life, but it is all a clouded mystery to her. Because of the intense pain she had been in, she has little memory of what she experienced in those ten days, and in days to come it would prove to be a continuing source of puzzlement to her. Although she had responded to us and spoken to the nurses and physicians while she was in Lahey's SICU, she tells me she now has almost no memory of what had happened to her for the entire period, between December 8 and December 18, when she had been experiencing excruciating pain.

On arriving at Dr. Nanda's office suite on the sixth floor, we are ushered in to an examining room where the physician assistant carefully examines Joanie's incision and pronounces that it is healing very nicely. She then proceeds to remove Joanie's sutures, working slowly and gently, as Todd, Janna, and I look on. It doesn't hurt her to have the sutures removed, as Joanie had feared, but just the same, she says, with a little smile in her voice, "I deserve some ice cream for this." Ice cream is, after all, her favorite food.

Afterwards, she doesn't feel like going out to a restaurant, so, to honor her tongue-in-cheek request, the four of us drive back home and have ice cream there.

Just as Joanie had felt strange emerging from the hospital, I am now beginning to feel some of those same sensations as I emerge from an existence that, over the past three weeks, was confined pretty much to Joanie's hospital room or our bedroom or family room at home, an existence that focused solely on her health. As she has become more engaged in life outside the sickroom, I am beginning to feel as if I, too, am emerging from some kind of underground world and coming out into the light. It is similar to how I felt many years earlier on coming home from the hospital the first and only time I had ever been a patient in one. Our experiences are akin, I think, to sensory deprivation and its aftermath.

Over the next weeks, I see the old Joanie beginning to emerge, but with pieces missing. She can't recall names of people and places that previously were second nature to her. It takes her over a week to get straight the names of the four prescription medications that she has to take daily now that she is out of the hospital. She will tell me, "Remember to call the pharmacy for my prescription," and then, an hour later, tell me again to call the pharmacy for her prescription. She tries some of the Monday *New York Times* puzzles—the easiest of the week of the *Times* crossword puzzles—that Todd has printed out for her, but even these give her some difficulty. She has to ask me if the word "adequate" is spelled with one "d" or two, and she writes "boarder" when she means "border."

It isn't just memory: there are pieces missing from her confidence, too. She is tentative in her actions, and she often looks to me for concurrence on even the simplest of decisions that, prior to her injury, she would have made on her own without a second thought. "Should I wear a scarf when we go outside today?" "What time should I get up for the nurse's visit tomorrow?"

It tugs at my heart to see her like this. I hope it won't last.

Wednesday, December 27

Joanie wakes up and has a hearty breakfast. Her appetite is returning, and, from other signs, I can tell that her sense of smell is, too (they are related, after all). Janna, Todd, or I walk her around the house at intervals to help her regain her strength and familiarity with her surroundings. The initial evaluations are now over, and the real work of the therapies aimed at rehabilitating her is to begin. Today, Joanie's rehabilitation starts to take on a pattern that will continue for the next several weeks: two or three visits almost every day from the nurse or rehabilitation therapists.

First nurse Nancy comes. She takes her blood pressure, pulse, and temperature (all are in the normal range) and asks her to rate her head pain on the 0 to 10 scale we have become so familiar with. Joanie rates it at about a 2 to 3. Good—her pain is way down.

Next to arrive is Tricia Reed, the physical therapist, who will work with Joanie over the coming weeks to help her regain her body strength, movement coordination, and balance, all of which are subpar.

Tricia tests Joanie by pushing her forcefully in various directions to see how well she keeps her balance. She watches her walk and do a few other movements. She then prescribes a set of exercises to strengthen her core muscles and improve her balance and endurance. Tricia instructs her carefully on how to do each exercise, warning her that she should stand in front of a kitchen counter while doing them, and only do them with a helper (me) behind her, in case she loses her balance. She has Joan rock back and forth alternately on each foot (the hardest exercise for her to do and still keep her balance). Another exercise consists of lifting each knee slowly, bringing it up as far as she can, then slowly placing it back down. In all, she gives her six or seven exercises like these to do, ten repetitions each, twice each day.

Tricia also instructs her on how to stand safely so as to avoid losing her balance. She warns her not to try too much too fast. Because our impatient patient is determined to return to normal as quickly as she can, I see that I will have to be Tricia's alter-ego to make sure that the patient doesn't try to forge past her current capabilities and end up getting frustrated and discouraged, or, worse, fall and re-injure herself.

Thursday, December 28
Joanie needs no encouragement from me to do the balance and strengthening exercises Tricia gave her. She is resolved to get back to her old self as quickly

as possible, no external motivation required. She does her exercise routine twice, as instructed, once in the morning and again in the afternoon.

Later this morning, Laurie Thibodeau, the occupational therapist, arrives. She had arranged on her previous visit that today she would see how Joanie handles showering. With the stitches removed, she can now get her head wet (although the physician assistant warned that she was not to scrub her incision site nor allow shampoo to get on it), so she is free to shower at last.

When it comes to falls, the bathroom is one of the most dangerous places in the home. Laurie wants to ensure that Joanie can handle standing in our shower stall and performing all the bends and turns necessary to shower herself. On Laurie's previous instruction, I had borrowed a shower chair for Joanie to use if she needed to sit down at any point while showering. When they come downstairs after the shower, Laurie reports that Joan didn't need the chair except to wash her feet. She reiterates that we should have a grab bar installed in our shower, and not just for Joanie during her rehabilitation. Given our ages, she says it wouldn't be a bad idea to have one, for if we don't need it now, it would be a good thing to have for the future.

Although she had received sponge baths during her two hospitalizations, and Janna had washed half of her hair a few days earlier, this was Joanie's first real, full shower and shampoo in four weeks. She comes back downstairs a very happy camper. From today on, she begins spending the better part of each day dressed and downstairs.

Shortly after the big shower event, Joan's brother, Paul, arrives from Albany, New York to visit her. He had wanted to come sooner, but we had waved him off because we felt, for one thing, that his making the three hour drive from Albany to see her might signal to Joanie that her condition was grave and so might alarm her. For another, we felt that there wasn't much Paul could do or say to his sister that would help her in the foggy state she was in while in the hospital. But after her discharge, she's made progress from day to day, and at this point there is no reason for Paul not to come.

We give Paul lunch from our ample stock of already prepared food that our friends and neighbors have brought us. Joanie and her brother talk afterward in our family room, Paul on the rocking chair and Joanie on the sofa.

"After getting Larry's e-mails, I looked up subdural hematoma on the Internet. This is a serious injury, Joanie. You could've died."

Joanie remains quiet but is visibly taken aback by Paul's comment. Neither Janna, nor Todd, nor I had ever discussed outright with her that her condition was potentially so serious.

Later, she tells me "Oh my God, I had no idea it was that bad. That was the first inkling I had that it was so critical."

The knowledge that she has sustained a life-threatening injury stays with Joanie as, in the weeks ahead, she begins to express the desire, ever more fervently, to return to normal and put all this behind her.

They talk some more, and by the time Paul leaves it is apparent that it did both him and his sister a lot of good to be together today. As she has begun to feel better, it helps her outlook to be doing normal things again. Paul feels much relieved to spend time, and talk, with his sister and see that she is coming out of the woods.

In the afternoon, Joanie has her first home visit with the person from Emerson Hospital Home Care who will be working with her to improve her cognitive functioning. During our initial meeting with her speech therapist, Debbie Elliott, we all agree that "speech therapist" is something of a misnomer. Debbie isn't going to be working solely on Joanie's speech; rather, she is going to address the cognitive impairment (thinking and reading mainly, and speech secondarily) that Joanie suffered as a result of her fall.

In this, Debbie's initial visit, they run through some reading and logic exercises as a way of evaluating just where Joanie stands in her cognitive functioning. Debbie points out ways that Joanie can deal with the deficits that show themselves. She tells Joanie, for example, "When you can't find the word you want to say, try describing what it is. Approaching it from a different standpoint, using different brain processes, will help you find the word. Or, if you are reading and come to a word that doesn't make sense, sound it out aloud as you look at it. This uses different brain processes, and that might help you recognize the word."

Debbie instructs the rest of the family, too. "When Joan's speech becomes hesitant because she cannot get a word out that she is trying to say, you should resist the natural urge to supply the word or finish her sentence for her. Only by working through the cognitive processes to find the word or words and get them out will Joanie be able to strengthen the neuronal connections that have been disrupted by the injury to her brain." Although Joanie's speech, reading, and logical processes are really only moderately subpar (considering how much worse they could have been) as a result of her injury, she still will have a lot of work to do to get them back to their previous levels.

Friday, December 29

The physical therapist comes and observes as Joanie does her exercise routine. The therapist again tests Joanie's strength and balance by pushing her at several strategic points on her body to see how well she retains or regains her balance. She remarks that the patient is making good, noticeable progress. Todd, Janna, and I have noticed it, too. We are impressed with the strides, both literal and figurative, Joanie is making, and we tell her that often, as much to reassure ourselves as to encourage her.

After the physical therapist leaves, Joan and I walk outside for a short distance. Except for our trip back to the Lahey Clinic to have her sutures removed, this is the first time Joanie has left our house since her discharge from Lahey. Holding my arm tightly, she walks slowly out of the house and down the two steps from our door to the front path. Arm-in-arm, we go only a short way down the street—not even as far as the place where she had fallen—and then return. As much as for the exercise and fresh air, I want this walk to make a statement that Joanie is improving, that she can get outside (even if not on her own yet), that she is getting back into the swing of things, and that, eventually, she will be walking on her own to the coffee shop.

In the afternoon, Nancy Carolus, the nurse, pays us a visit. She, too, says that Joanie is doing fine physically— better than expected given the seriousness of her injury.

After she leaves, one of the regulars from our crowd at Boston Bean House, Denise Shea, shows up at our door with homemade soup and rolls for us. I ask Joanie if she feels up to seeing her, and when she says she does, I invite Denise in. They spend a little time chatting. Seeing the familiar face of one of the Boston Bean crowd and conversing with someone other than her family and her rehabilitation therapists means another step back to normality.

The remainder of the day is bittersweet. Todd is leaving tomorrow to fly back to California. He has been with us for nine days, and for those nine days, our entire family has been together to rally around Joan. That, I am convinced, accounts for a good bit of the progress she has made up to this point.

This evening, I send my first e-mail update since before Christmas. It reads, in part:

> *Joan has been home from the hospital for a little over a week now and is progressing well. She's been getting dressed and spending each day downstairs, and her appetite has returned and she's eating well. She had her stitches removed earlier this week and was very happy to be rid of them. That was her first and only time she's been out of the house since getting out of the hospital, and she still is reluctant to talk on the phone, but overall, she's slowly getting back to normal activities . . . .*
>
> *All of [her rehabilitation therapists]—to a person—have remarked how much Joanie has improved over the short time she's been out of the hospital. Each day, we (Todd, Janna, and I) can see that she is noticeably better than the day before in all her functions.*

Getting out of the hospital made the holiday week special for all of us. Janna has been staying here over the holidays until she has to return to work early next week. Todd has been here for a little over a week and will leave to fly back to San Francisco tomorrow (Saturday). Having both Todd and Janna here for the holidays was a joy for both Joanie and me and has helped speed her recovery and make things easier for us. No surprise—we'll be looking forward to a happier, healthier [year to come]. Happy New Year to you all.

Saturday, December 30

I wake up to take Todd to Logan Airport for his early morning flight back to San Francisco. Joanie has insisted on being awakened, despite the early hour, to say goodbye to him before we leave for the airport. On the way there, I tell Todd how much his visit has meant to his Mom, but I know he already knows that and was glad he came in when he did.

The rest of the day is quiet—no rehabilitation therapists. I run some needed errands after I return home from dropping Todd off, and then Janna, Joanie, and I just laze around the house until bedtime.

Sunday, December 31

Whether it is the end of a bad year (really, only the last month of it has been bad), the departure of our children (Todd yesterday, Janna this evening), or beginning to get enough of her faculties back to reflect more on her injury, Joanie doesn't show much initiative or motivation today. She watches the New England Patriots football game on television with Janna and me, after which Janna returns to her apartment to prepare to go out with friends this evening (it is New Year's Eve, after all).

Joanie does her physical and cognitive exercises, and then we walk around outside, this time farther than our initial walk a couple of days ago. In fact, today's walk takes us past the place on Robert Road where she had fallen four weeks before. She has no noticeable reaction when we pass it.

For the remainder of the day—and this really concerns me—she sits inertly on our sofa watching a marathon of reruns of the television comedy show *Ugly Betty*. Hours and hours of it.

"What's bothering you, Joanie?"

"I'm depressed, Lar. This really shouldn't have happened to me. Here we are young for our age, we did things to feel and be healthy, and here it is New Year's Eve and something as stupid as my falling has thrown a wrench into all that." She goes on: "And you know how you see people on *America's Funniest Home Videos* doing all sorts of stupid things and falling all over the place, and they don't get hurt. Here I was doing something healthful, and I get a severe head injury."

I can understand where she is coming from. In fact, she is expressing my attitude about the whole chain of events, as well.

I do my best to draw her out more and listen to her plaint. There is not much more I can do other than be there for her and listen to her. The very idea of suffering a traumatic brain injury while exercising to keep oneself fit is, we both clearly feel, worse than ironic. It is unfair.

People who suffer from catastrophic injury or illness often feel this way. Why me? What did I do to deserve this? Everything was going along fine, then this. Why did it have to happen? Listening to Joanie, reflecting her feelings, being there physically and emotionally for her is what I can do to help her work through her frustration and help drive her recovery. I often feel this is inadequate in the face of these overwhelming events, but in the end, I believe it is the best thing I can do.

Although it is New Years Eve, Joanie goes up to bed at eight o'clock. In recent years, she and I have seldom stayed up to see the new year in anyway. We both don't like crowds all that much, or forcing ourselves to stay awake for what is, in some ways, an artificial-feeling holiday. But this year, it isn't just weariness that sends her up to bed so early. She is in a poor frame of mind.

Monday, January 1
The dawning of a new year isn't accompanied by much of a change in Joanie's mood. She is still depressed

and not showing much initiative. Since there are no rehabilitation therapists scheduled today, Joanie doesn't even have that to look forward to. On the other hand, we discover to our surprise that Janna came back to our house early in the morning while we were both still asleep.

Janna inherited our lack of enthusiasm for New Year's Eve celebrations. She had gone with friends last evening to Boston's First Night celebration and, as in previous years, she was underwhelmed. On her way back to her apartment in the city, she observed two men about her age in the same subway car, obviously intoxicated. One of them proceeded to get sick in the train car, and the other proceeded to urinate in the doorway of the car. Seeing that, she decided to pack up some clothes at her apartment and flee the city for our house in the quiet, subdued suburbs.

Janna's presence helps lift Joanie's mood slightly, but only slightly. She remains lethargic and shows little initiative for the rest of the day.

Tuesday, January 2

Laurie Thibodeau comes, and without any prompting from me about Joanie's frame of mind, the occupational therapist says that Joanie can and should start doing more of her normal activities, beginning with preparing her own breakfast and lunch each day. She tells her that the more she engages in her pre-injury activities, the

sooner she will get back to normal. That is all Joanie
has to hear—she wants nothing more than to get back to
being the person she was before her injury, and I suspect
that her feelings of depression are due in good measure
to her frustration at not being there yet.

On reflection, I think that the family's actions—
especially mine—may have slowed her progress
toward achieving normality, adding to the frustration
and depression she is feeling. In the days immediately
following her return home from the hospital, Todd,
Janna, and I waited on her hand and foot. It wasn't
because she was confined to bed or that she demanded
it. It was because she was still stunned at everything
that had happened to her and didn't have the energy,
drive, motivation, or confidence to do much on her
own. Because she was still weak physically and in a fog
mentally, the rest of us went to bat to do the things she
would normally have done herself. Todd and I did the
food shopping, I served her breakfast and lunch, Todd
and Janna took care of dinners, and Janna changed the
sheets and towels and did the laundry and the many
other home chores Todd and I left undone.

Our aim was to keep the house running as it usually
did so that when Joan emerged from her cocoon, she
would be back in an environment that was functioning
normally. In all the bustle of activity that we undertook
to keep house and home together, we failed to recognize,
because the changes were gradual, that each day Joanie

was becoming stronger physically and clearer mentally, and that she could begin to fend for herself more. We would have to stop treating her as an invalid.

Laurie also proposes that, on her next appointment two days later, Joanie should prepare dinner while Laurie observes. This will allow the occupational therapist to assess how well her patient engages in planning and completing a sequence of tasks, such as those required to plan and then prepare a meal, and to see how safely she carries them out. In preparation for the meal-making exercise, Laurie has Joanie decide what she is going to make for that meal and then check on what ingredients she already has at hand so that she can compose a shopping list for those items that are needed.

Joanie is still having trouble with words, finding them and expressing them orally and, in reading, recognizing them. This is driven home when she and Laurie go through our pantry cupboard to see what ingredients are already there to use for the planned dinner, a shrimp stir fry. Joanie tells Laurie that she usually prepares the dish using a sauce Trader Joe's supermarket sells, but she can't remember the name of it to put on the shopping list. She rummages through the kitchen cupboard looking to see if she has a jar of that particular sauce, and then, holding something in her hand, tells Laurie she can't come up with it.

"What's that you're holding?" Laurie asks. It's a jar of the Cuban Mojito sauce Joanie had been looking for, but even with it in her hand, she fails to recognize it.

Wednesday, January 3

Tricia arrives for Joan's physical therapy appointment with two new exercises aimed at strengthening her hip muscles. She compliments her on her progress in regaining more of her strength and balance. When Joanie answers with the rejoinder "But why don't I feel normal, and when will I be completely normal again?" Tricia tells her that *total* healing, with all of the parts (physical, cognitive, emotional) functioning in synch again, will likely take a matter of months.

"The brain is an intricate mechanism controlling all these body functions, and when it is severely jolted, as yours was, it'll take time for all the connections to go back to how they worked together, as an integral whole, before," the physical therapist explains. "And sometimes, they don't get back completely to how they worked before."

I don't think Joanie likes Tricia's answer. But I do think that as more and more people tell her she is going to get there eventually ("there" being back to normal, back to her old self), it is beginning to sink in that it will take more time.

In reality, she is progressing on all fronts faster than anyone (except herself) expected. This is not just my opinion, but the opinion of the nurse and the three therapists who are working with her. Granted, their professional training calls for them to be encouraging and cheerful, but I can tell that they truly are impressed with how fast and how well she is progressing. The only person who is not so impressed is Joanie herself. Her will to recover *completely* is strong and eager, and she wants to be back to normal in a matter of days—not weeks or months. But it is beginning to sink in even with Joanie that maybe those other people are right, and she will have to be a more patient patient.

In the afternoon, Debbie Elliott arrives to give Joanie exercises to help her regain more of her cognitive functioning. One is a "fill in the letters" exercise where Debbie shows her words in various categories that have some letters missing, and Joanie has to fill in the missing letters. For example, in the "stores" category, she is shown words like _ro_ery and h_r_war_ and she is to complete the words (*grocery* and *hardware*). Because reading smoothly involves recognizing the general idea of words, not mentally sounding out each letter to conceptualize each word, this exercise is meant to facilitate Joanie's readiness to "get" the idea of each word when several letters are missing and to fill in the missing letters once she's got it. Joanie does the exercises deliberately and slowly, but, on the whole, accurately.

As if to reinforce the point that Joanie is getting back in shape, our friend, Mary Nadwairski, stops by this evening to see Joanie for the first time since her injury. I meet Mary in our breezeway, and we talk there before going into the house itself. She asks me apprehensively, "What can I expect, Larry? It sounds so awful what Joanie's had to endure."

"She's doing remarkably well," I tell her, "She's not the same old Joanie, yet, but she's coming along. But see for yourself when you go in."

When Mary goes inside and sees Joanie sitting on our family room sofa, tears pour from Mary's eyes. Some months later, she confides in me that her tears were from a mixture of joy at seeing that Joan looked better than she expected and sadness at how vulnerable, still, she looked sitting there. That encapsulates Joanie's progress up to this point: she's not as good as she was before her accident, but she's noticeably better than she was right after it.

Thursday, January 4

Around noon, as we are sitting in our family room, someone rings our doorbell. Joanie jumps up to get her Boston Red Sox cap to put on as I answer the door. Her cap has been the constant device she uses to hide her strange haircut and scalp scar whenever someone outside the family is present. She has always been conscious of how her hair looks, and now with it looking so abnormal, she is ultra self-conscious about it.

Dawn, who runs Boston Bean, is at the door with a Boston Bean House CARE package for us: two of the sandwiches we regularly order whenever we have lunch there, two coffees, and some luscious pastries. It's a surprise, and a nice one, to see her (after all, Boston Bean House doesn't normally deliver to Acton). Dawn is someone we would see regularly at least several times a week, and now neither of us has seen her for over four weeks. We invite her in and ask her to bring us up to date on what is happening at the shop and with our friends at the Bean. We especially thank her for the basket garden she and the gang from the Bean sent Joanie while she was in Lahey. There are hugs all around as Dawn leaves.

Joan is very self-conscious about her hair during Dawn's visit, as she has been with the few visitors who've come to see her since her hospitalization. She had intended to make an appointment in early December to have her hair cut, but the accident delayed that. Now, her head had been shaved on one side in preparation for the operation—without much attention paid to matters of hair style—while the other side has kept growing. With almost no hair on the left side of her head and the hair at the back of her head long, Todd, Janna, and I refer to her new, unwanted hair style as "the mullet."

Joan and I go out for a walk around the neighborhood after Dawn leaves. Joan, of course, wears her hat, more to cover her hair than to keep her head warm (she actually hates wearing hats). Each walk we

take is a little longer than the one before. Certainly
Joanie's stride is stronger and more rapid, I notice, to
the point that I now have to struggle to keep up with her
pace (just as I did before her accident).

As we start back up our driveway after our walk
around the neighborhood, two of our friends from
the Boston Bean House crowd, Linda Watskin and
Dorothy Leland, drive up. They have come with a
package of food they intended to leave at our door. They
are surprised to see Joanie up and about outside (and
walking at close to her normal speed). We invite them
in. They clearly are overjoyed to see Joanie looking
so well. They have not seen her since her accident,
and I suspect that they, like Mary the day before, were
expecting the worst. While Linda and Dorothy visit,
Joanie keeps her cap on, even inside the house.

Laurie comes late this afternoon for the dinner-
making exercise. She watches as Joanie slices the
vegetables, heats the skillet, cooks the shrimp and
vegetables, and finally adds the Cuban Mojito sauce to
the stir fry. It fills the house with piquant aromas. As the
meal is cooking, Laurie pronounces, "Joanie, you did
the sequencing and preparation very well (and safely).
You're all ready to resume making dinner regularly."

"Oh, great, now that I'm progressing, I have to start
cooking again?" Joanie rejoinders. Her little joke shows
that her verve is starting to make a comeback.

But in the back of her mind, she isn't quite ready to feel normal. Her first followup CT scan since her hospitalization is scheduled for tomorrow, and the first followup appointment with Dr. Nanda is scheduled for next Monday. She has been rigorously and conscientiously adhering to her medication and exercise regime with the expectation that this will speed her recovery, but Joanie wants so much to hear the words from the neurosurgeon that everything is "okay inside my brain" before she will allow herself to feel okay. There is nothing to do but wait for that pronouncement.

Friday, January 5

The CT scan is scheduled for eight a.m., so we leave for Lahey at seven o'clock to allow plenty of time, in the face of rush hour traffic, to get there punctually. While we are on our way there, a Saab passes us on the highway. She stares at the car's nameplate as it passes by and then asks me, incredulously, "There's a car called a Saab?" It is as if she were seeing it for the first time, even though one of her friends had recently bought a Saab, and even though we have driven past a Saab dealership near our home many times before.

On arriving at the Lahey Clinic's lobby, Joanie again marvels at how big and busy a place it is. We go down to the CT scan unit, where she is signed in and given a brief medical history questionnaire to complete. Pretty soon she is called in for her scan, and I settle in to reading a magazine while I wait. I am taken aback by how quickly Joanie returns from her scan; apparently, having an appointment for it makes things go ultra-smoothly. We still have to wait while they check the images to be sure that they are comprehensive and complete. They are, so we are free to leave. We stop at a nearby Starbuck's for coffee and a scone and drive home (with Joanie in the "safe position" in the center of the rear seat).

After we arrive home, Tricia Reed comes for her scheduled eleven a.m. appointment. She says that Joan is progressing so well in her physical recovery that she is going to discharge her next week from home-based physical therapy. This decision is based both on Joan's current physical condition as well as Tricia's assessment that Joanie will soon no longer be considered "homebound." Even though Joanie does not trust herself to drive, that is not a consideration in determining her status as homebound or not. Once she is no longer considered homebound, her health insurance will no longer cover home visits. Tricia points out, however, that Joan is eligible for outpatient physical therapy should she feel a need for it.

She writes out a memo for us to give to Dr. Nanda summarizing Joan's status and progress: "Will be discharged in 1-2 weeks from homecare P.T. . . . She has very minimal weakness in her prox. leg strength, good safety awareness and independent at home." She recommends no further outpatient physical therapy.

Debbie Elliott arrives later in the afternoon for speech therapy, and she and Joan talk about her progress. They work on more cognitive functioning exercises.

Since Joanie is so self-conscious about her hair, I urge her to make an appointment to have her hair cut the following week. I know that she wants to wait until she has had her appointment with Dr. Nanda this coming Monday—in order to be sure that she is *really* returning to normal—before she takes that step. But if she waits until then, she might not be able to get an appointment until the week after that. I prevail, and she telephones for a hair appointment. Joanie tells Tish, the beautician, about her surgery and how strange her hair now looks as a result.

"Have you ever cut anyone's hair who's been in the same situation as me?" Joanie asks. She thinks that her predicament—facing others with such an uneven haircut—is unusual, but Tish assures her that it is not as unusual as Joanie thinks. She has dealt with several women whose hair had been shaved for medical or surgical reasons, Tish says. "So you shouldn't worry about how it's going to come out," she assures her.

Joan had been invited to a baby shower on Sunday for Mei-Lyn Kingsley, a neighbor expecting her first child toward the end of the month. The shower is being organized by a couple of other neighbors. Joanie still doesn't feel self-confident, and she was apprehensive that being in a crowd of people might tire her out, but she decided she would go so long as Janna would accompany her. Besides, she reasoned, since the shower was going to be just down the street and mainly neighbors would be there, how badly could it turn out?

In the evening, Janna comes to our house to spend the weekend. Mother and daughter make plans to go out together tomorrow to buy a shower gift and then, the day after, to go together to the baby shower.

Susanne Fuller, who is hosting the shower, sends me an e-mail asking what she can do to make Joanie's first time out among a group of other people more comfortable. I read Joanie the e-mail, and she tells me to answer Susanne that "the best thing she [Susanne] could do would be not to make a fuss over me. I want it to be Mei-Lyn's event, not mine." I also tell Susanne in my reply e-mail that, since the shower will be the first time in about two months that Joanie will be among more than four people at one time, it might prove to be tiring or overwhelming for her. "If she leaves early," I write, "I don't want you to be offended or worried."

Saturday, January 6

While we wait for Janna to wake up, Joanie sits and works on one of the *Times* Monday crossword puzzles Todd had left for her. I can see that while she is doing it more quickly than just a few days before, she is still not zipping through it as fast as she normally would.

Once Janna wakes up, Joanie takes a shower and washes her hair. I remark how nice her hair is looking now that she has begun to be able to wash at least that part of it that doesn't have an incision in it. Despite my encouraging remarks, she still puts on a Boston Red Sox cap to hide her hair before she leaves with Janna to shop for the baby shower gift. They return a good couple of hours later, having shopped for a gift at two stores and then stopped for coffee. Joanie enthusiastically shows me the little pink outfit and silver piggy bank they have selected for Mei-Lyn and John's baby (they knew it would be a girl), and then she wraps the gifts.

I ask Joanie how she tolerated her foray into the outside world. "Everything went well, and I'm beginning to feel better," she answers. It's beginning to look that way to me, too.

Sunday, January 7

Judy Gettig, Joanie's friend, has been away in Florida with her husband since before Christmas. They returned yesterday, and Judy is anxious to see Joanie, as the last time she saw her was when she was in grave condition in the Surgical Intensive Care Unit at Lahey. Shortly before the baby shower is to start, Judy comes over to our house. She and Joan hug warmly, and Judy holds her friend at arm's length to take a good look at her. "How good you look," she tells Joanie.

Wearing her Boston Red Sox cap, Joan leaves with Judy and Janna for the short walk down the street to Susanne's house. I half-expect Joanie to return home within an hour or two of leaving. She still acts a little slow in her response to others' conversation, and being at the shower among more people than she has been with since before her accident, I expect that the strain of following conversation and participating in it would tire her out quickly. Yet she stays almost three hours. When she returns home, she tells me, "That was something of a strain to be among all those people, but although I feel a little tired, I wasn't overwhelmed."

Apparently, Susanne had clued in the other baby shower attendees (mostly other women from our neighborhood) about Joanie's wish not to be fussed over, for Joanie reports that other than some passing questions about how she was feeling, no one talked much about her accident and subsequent course in the hospital. Before and after the opening of the shower gifts, Joan, Janna, and Judy spent most of their time in the Fullers' family room, where there was a smaller crowd than the one milling in the kitchen.

Tonight is also my first night back among a crowd of people since Joanie's accident. I had missed the December Board meeting of the Acton Historical Society, but, since Janna is here with Joanie, I feel that it will be all right to attend the society's January general meeting.

I am glad that we both have something to occupy our minds this weekend. It has kept us from worrying about what the neurosurgeon's verdict might be when we meet with him tomorrow.

Monday, January 8

This is D-Day—Joanie's long awaited first followup appointment with her neurosurgeon since being discharged from the Lahey Clinic hospital. Here is where the all-important messages would be delivered: about the most recent CT scan of her brain; about what she could now do, or no longer do anymore; about whether her eagerly anticipated return to normality is going to be a reality.

Janna leaves our house early to go to her teaching job, after which she plans to stop by her apartment. Joanie talks to her by telephone later in the morning. Todd telephones us from San Francisco. We both talk to him about Joanie's progress and what lies ahead today. He remarks to Joanie, "I notice how much better your command of the English language is compared with last week." He then goes on to tell us (as he usually does in our weekly phone calls) how his week went, and he wishes his mother well at her appointment.

We leave for Dr. Nanda's office in the Lahey Clinic, arriving a little before our one o'clock appointment. Immediately after checking in at the desk, we are called in to one of the examining rooms in the office suite, where the nurse asks Joanie questions about her medications, pain, and any problems she might still be having. Joanie reports no major problems on any of these fronts. The nurse then takes Joanie's blood pressure and pulse. We wait some time after those preliminaries are over for Dr. Nanda to come into the examining room, and while we do we nervously pass the time talking about Joanie's progress since being in the hospital and what has happened to her while she was there (much of which is but a vague memory to her).

"Let's get right away to the news you've been waiting for," Dr. Nanda says as he sweeps into the room and greets us. He pulls up all the earlier CT scan images on the computer monitor in the examining room, along with the most recent one. "This is a very normal looking brain," he says of the latest scan, "Very symmetrical. Here's a tiny residual area of blood in your left temporal area," he says, showing us a slightly darkened spot on the scan image that looks like a black-and-white photo of a meteorite hitting the moon and kicking up dust. He indicates that, first, the dark spot is so much smaller than what appeared on previous CT scans, and, second, he expects even the small amount of blood it represents to be reabsorbed by the time Joanie has her next CT scan next month.

To show us how well things are looking inside her skull, he points out by comparison the CT image of Joanie's brain that was done the day before her operation (the image that caused him to decide not even to wait until the next morning to perform the operation when scheduled, but to do it immediately). He points to where, on the left side of her skull in that earlier image, fluid had accumulated to such an extent that it was displacing the midline of her brain by a considerable twelve millimeters, compressing and deforming it. Clicking back to her most recent CT scan, he then shows us how the left and right lateral ventricles (natural fluid-filled cavities in each cerebral hemisphere) now show up as symmetrical, horseshoe-shaped areas on either side of the midline in her now-normal-looking, now-symmetrical brain. Then—clicking back to her December 14 pre-surgery CT scan—he points out how the excess fluid surrounding her brain then had compressed one of the ventricle spaces to the point where it could barely be seen on the scan.

Then Joanie asks the question that has been burning in her mind ever since she came home from her hospital stay at Lahey: "When will I be back to normal?" Dr. Nanda forecasts that she will be at "about 95 percent in another month. Physically and medically, you've recovered very well, but subtle cognitive things will take longer—maybe six months to a year." He concurs with the Emerson Hospital Home Care workers' opinions that there seems to be little further need for physical or occupational therapy and that any further rehabilitation efforts should be directed toward fully recovering her cognitive functioning.

Joanie then peppers him with a raft of questions we had written down beforehand to make sure we wouldn't forget them, and I record his answers on a pad I brought:

"When will my head pain be completely gone?"

"Probably in a few weeks."

"What do I need to do to ensure that my blood sodium level is maintained at normal levels?"

"Nothing—it seems to be stabilized."

"What special care do I need to take for my incision site?"

"For at least a month, don't rub it hard, and keep harsh chemicals away from it."

"How about for the burr hole?"

"Nothing—it will knit together on its own, maybe leaving a small depression showing in your skin."

"How long should I continue taking the medications?"

"Start tailing off the pain medication, but continue taking the preventive anti-seizure medication for another month."

"When can I resume taking my normal daily nutritional supplements?"

"Immediately, except for Vitamin E and low-dose aspirins because they cause the blood to thin."

"When can I resume walking, driving, bike riding?"

"As you feel up to it, except wait until the weather improves in the spring to resume biking, just because some of the roads are still icy."

"What activities should I not do?"

"Don't do anything that would subject your head to shaking or shock."

Dr. Nanda tells us he would like Joan to have another CT scan followed by an appointment with him in about a month. Big smiles start to creep across each of our faces, and Joanie and I grasp hands and give each other a heartfelt squeeze. Victory is in sight.

We leave his office elated and relieved. She has heard the news directly from her neurosurgeon's mouth that her injury is healing and that her brain is looking normal. It is what Joanie had been hoping with all her heart to hear before she would allow herself to believe that, yes, she will eventually recover and be normal again.

We have lunch at the nearby Dandelion Green restaurant to celebrate the verdict. As we eat, she comments that this is the first time she has been to a restaurant in about a month and a half. In fact, it is the first time Joanie and I have been out in a public place together (hospital and physician appointments don't count) in that same period of time.

"We're reentering the land of the living," I tell her.

On the way home from the restaurant, I think to myself that the most recent CT scan of her brain that I had been looking at earlier in Dr. Nanda's office was the loveliest picture of Joanie I have ever seen.

Three more milestones await us over the course of the week.

Tuesday, January 9

Joanie and I talked the week before about whether or not she would be okay being all alone if I were to keep a long-standing appointment for my annual eye exam. We had agreed that she could manage it so long as I had my cell phone with me. Today will be the first time she has been alone since before the accident, and it is with some trepidation that I leave her, but at the same time, I feel that her being home alone will be another confirmation for her that she is getting back to normal. Thank goodness for cell phones, I think, as I leave the house.

I keep the appointment and then do a few errands that I had been putting off. I return home early in the afternoon. Joanie has managed fine in my absence, further reinforcing in her mind Dr. Nanda's assessment that she is, indeed, returning to normal.

When Debbie Elliott, her cognitive therapist, comes, she asks how the appointment yesterday with the neurosurgeon had gone. Joanie tells her about it and relays to her Dr. Nanda's concurrence that she should continue cognitive therapy for at least a month longer.

Seeing Joanie interacting with the therapists and friends who came to the house over the previous few days, I can see that some of her vivacity is returning. Her depression of the week before is now a thing of the past. She smiles more, some of her old verve is back, and she is becoming more self-assured, although she still has a way to go in all these departments.

By prior arrangement, Janna comes to our house this evening to stay with Joanie so that I can attend a meeting I need to go to. Things really do seem to be getting back to normal, and so, when I return after the meeting, I compose the last e-mail report on Joanie's status that I will send to our friends and relatives. I let them know about her overall progress, the good report we received from the neurosurgeon yesterday, and how significant their support has been to us. The e-mail concludes:

> *Now that things are looking up, this will be my last update report to you. Joanie, Todd, Janna, and I have been buoyed by the caring and concern you all have shown toward us throughout this whole ordeal. Your e-mails, messages, cards, letters, flowers, good wishes, and all the other expressions of your love and friendship over the past six weeks have made a world of difference in Joanie's recovery. We have no doubt that it has helped her get to this point as rapidly as she has, and we are so very grateful to you.*

Wednesday, January 10

Another day, another milestone: this is the day of Joanie's appointment to have her hair cut at Tish's. By now, the hair on the left side of her scalp has grown enough so that her incision scar, while still visible, is starting to be covered over by her hair. Only if I look closely can I see the scar through her hair. Yet the hair on her right side has continued to grow, too, providing an overall lopsided effect. Before she left to go back to her job and apartment, Janna discussed with Joanie what might be done with her hair at the beauty parlor, but they came to no conclusion, as neither of them had had that particular styling problem up to that point in their lives. With some apprehension on Joanie's part, we leave to drive to the beauty salon.

I wait in a chair and look around the neat, sleek salon at Joanie and the other women having their hair tended to. Joanie and the beautician consult about her hair and decide what to do with it. Tish gives her a very short cut in the back and on her right side. The resulting cut doesn't quite even out the right and left sides of her hair, but it looks a lot better. She no longer has "the mullet."

Nancy Carolus comes over for her final nursing visit this afternoon. She notices Joanie's hair right away and remarks enthusiastically, "Well, that makes a noticeable difference in how you look." She doesn't even bother to take Joanie's vital signs. She can see how much she has improved from the first time she had visited her at home two and a half weeks ago, and she tells her she is discharging her from her care with this visit. As she leaves, we thank Nancy for all she has done.

Janna comes back to stay with us tonight. When she arrives, she ponders Joanie's new haircut for a while and then says, "You know, Mom, if you put some gel down the middle, you could spike it up into a Mohawk." The absurdity of picturing Joanie with that particular hair style gives us all a good laugh.

Liz Gabel, another friend of ours, drops by. She has not seen Joanie since the accident. They sit and talk about how Joanie is doing, their respective families, and how they spent the holidays. Later, Liz tells me (as Mary Nadwairski had done) how vulnerable Joanie appeared as she sat on the corner of our sofa talking with her.

Thursday, January 11

The return to Boston Bean House is the next milestone event. A couple of weeks before, Denise, one of the Bean regulars, told me she wanted to do something special to welcome Joanie on her first day back— whenever that might be. "Nothing elaborate," she said, "just something low-key that wouldn't make Joanie feel too much in the spotlight."

Joanie never liked being the center of attention, which Denise knew from our years of contact at the Bean. With the positive report from Dr. Nanda earlier

this week under our belt, I phoned Denise to tell her
that I selected Thursday morning for Joanie's "official"
return to the Bean. I now tell Joanie about it so that she
won't be taken aback at today's welcoming reception.

We still can't walk into Maynard yet—that will have
to wait a while. Joan (wearing a cap, of course), Janna,
and I drive to the Bean. When we enter, we see a table
with a yellow tablecloth spread out over it, topped by
a vase of hydrangeas and a sign reading: "Reserved for
Joanie Kerpelman and guests." Denise, Dorothy, Linda,
and Ben are seated at other tables as we come in and,
with hugs all around, we sit at the "table of honor" they
had prepared for us. Dawn and young Eli are working
behind the counter, and they, too, come over to greet us.
Everyone says how much they missed Joanie and how

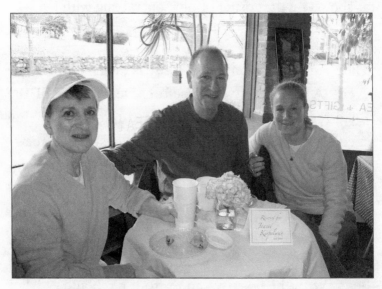

At our special table on "Return to the Bean" day.

the Bean just hasn't seemed the same in the six weeks we've been gone. They also jokingly point out how the books that were arrayed on the bookshelves of the coffee shop for patrons to read have gotten all out of order during Joanie's long absence.

We relax over our beverages, kibbitz with the other regulars, and enjoy the ambiance. "It's nice to feel normal," Joanie says several times that morning. "Just sitting here and having coffee, and looking out the window at the cars going by makes me feel that I've really come back." We stay for a couple of hours, but before we leave, Joanie the librarian sets about putting the bookshelves back in order. Dawn insists that we take lunches back with us, on the house.

Friday, January 12

Today we reach one last milestone. Joanie has three rehabilitation appointments: with Tricia, the physical therapist, Debbie, the cognitive therapist, and Laurie, the occupational therapist. For Tricia and Laurie, it is to be their last sessions with Joanie, as her physical recovery has progressed to the point that they believe there is not much more they can do for her.

Joan has done as much to help herself recover as the therapists did for her—motivation that the therapists applauded her for all through the weeks. She has been very driven, determined to do all she could to get herself back in shape as quickly as she could. What seemed to motivate her more than anything else over these past few weeks was her desire to return to her normal activities, and especially to resume walking to Maynard every day. Though that will still be several weeks into the future, Tricia and Laura have done all they could to help her get to that point.

Debbie comes and works with Joanie on some more advanced cognitive exercises than they had previously done. One of them challenges Joanie's ability to sequence things logically. It consists of sentences of a story that are out of order, and Joanie has to put them in the correct logical sequence to tell the story coherently. She does most of them correctly, except for one, Debbie tells her. When Joanie explains the reasons she sequenced it the way she did (which was supposedly incorrect), Debbie agrees that the story would also make sense the way Joanie has structured it.

At the end of the session, Debbie indicates that she will continue cognitive therapy with Joanie for a while more, but since she will no longer be considered homebound in a week or two, she will have to transfer her to an outpatient therapist at that point. Debbie supplies the name and contact information of an outpatient cognitive therapist, whom Joanie later calls to arrange for an initial appointment.

Joanie wants to send thank you notes to our friends and relatives. This evening, I collaborate with her in drafting a general letter she can tailor to each of the thirty or so people who had brought food and flowers or sent encouraging notes. She writes each one out slowly and laboriously by hand, and it takes her the next several days to complete them all.

Saturday, January 13

It has been six weeks to the day of Joanie's accident, but an end of some kind seems to be in sight. We don't mark the day as a momentous one, but in retrospect, it is the end of a week that has seen incredible progress.

Ruth Flynn, Joan's close friend from the quilting guild, has not visited her since the accident. She stops over this morning to see Joan. Knowing Joanie's liking for scones, she brings some with her, and they settle down to have scones and coffee. I assume Ruth will stay an hour at most, but they get to talking, and pretty soon an hour has passed and they are still talking. Another hour passes, and they are still at it. After three hours, Ruth says her goodbyes and leaves. I expect to find Joanie exhausted by the visit, but instead she is positively buoyed by it.

Joanie and I take a walk around the neighborhood and talk about what a long, strange journey these last six weeks have been, made even stranger by Joanie's inability to remember a good ten days of it. It has been an arduous trip, with ups and downs, highs and lows, and memorable moments and many Joanie can't remember as hard as she tries. In that six week period, she had sustained a terrible injury that sapped her strength, assaulted her confidence, and impaired her memory. In those six weeks, she suffered through three emergency room visits, two hospitalizations, and one brain surgery. During that period, she experienced an enforced isolation from friends and much of the outside world. But in those six weeks, too, she has completed the recommended course of physical and occupational therapy at home, the nurse has discharged her, and, most of all, her neurosurgeon has said her brain is looking normal.

Although she is to continue with her cognitive therapy on an outpatient basis, she is well on her way to recovery. She has begun to find the pieces missing and to put them back into place.

7

AFTEREFFECTS

THE BIGGEST BATTLE is over, but the war continues. Although she is no longer receiving home visits from her physical or occupational therapists, Joanie continues on her own the balance, coordination, and strengthening exercises they have given her. Every morning, without fail, I hear her chanting "One, two, three, four"—up to thirty-five—as she does her high-step exercise, her "wiggle walk," and the other physical exercises she has been given for her rehabilitation, all with five pound weights strapped to her ankles. Her "wiggle walk," as she calls it, is comical to watch, as she holds onto the kitchen counter for safety and sidles her way to one side by placing her left leg sideways behind her, followed by moving her right leg to the right in front of her, then the left leg to the same side in front of her, and so on to snake along the counter. She has continued these exercises even past the point in time that it was recommended she continue them. She is a very motivated camper, determined to build her strength so that one day—soon, I could tell—she would be able to resume her walks all the way to Boston Bean House, a mile and a half away, and back.

Winter

All through the winter, Joanie continues to have little memory of that period from December 8, two days after her release from Emerson Hospital, to December 18, two days after her neurosurgery at the Lahey Clinic. She calls it her "blank out period."

"I have almost no recollection of what happened then," she relates. "I don't remember being taken in an ambulance back to Emerson or how I ended up in Lahey. I do remember being in the intensive care unit at Lahey and trying to remove the dressing that was on my head—it must have been after surgery—and either Janna or the nurse crying out 'What are you doing?' and stopping me. I remember being sat down in a chair at some point during that time. But that's about it for that whole time."

Going into February, she doesn't want to know what had happened to her during her "blank out period," and I don't push any details on her. I view it as her brain's protective mechanism in the face of the trauma it endured. I assume that she will start asking me more about that time when she feels comfortable doing so. It is strange, from my vantage point, that she has almost no memory of those ten days, because she did talk to the nurses, physicians, Janna, and me during that time. We had no idea then how little of it her body and brain would let her remember afterward.

Her brain needs a rest, and Janna and I figure that she does not need to relive, until she is ready, that highly traumatic period of her life when she was in such constant, deep pain. Once she starts asking, Janna or I feed her the details she asks for, helping her fill in those missing pieces as best we can. When we supply them to her, she is taken aback at the extent of her injury and debilitation and at the seriousness of the surgery that was performed on her. And while she begins to say it less frequently, she still proclaims her mantra as it all starts to come back, "Of all the stupid things to have happen to me."

She also begins to read from our e-mail archive the e-mails I had sent out informing our friends and relatives what was happening with her and the e-mails they sent in reply. It is a way for her to take in that troubling information at her own pace. These e-mails— over a hundred of them—from our friends are touching, and Joanie can read only so many of them at one time before she has to take a break, emotionally drained. The e-mails, too, help her recall what had happened to her after that first hospitalization, yet the experience of bringing to the fore all her pain and suffering weighs on her, and it is a long, long time before she can work her way through reading them all.

The totality of the information she learns—about her brain injury, her treatment in the hospital, her neurosurgery, our friends' responses to it—strikes her with a mixture of awe (that it could have happened to her without being able to remember most of it) and frustration (that it could have happened to her at all). There are pieces missing that she is only now beginning to fill in.

The details of the accident itself—of that terrible day on December 2 when her head came in contact with the asphalt and all the pain, the initial treatments she received, the first hospitalization—these remain vivid to her. She occasionally experiences flashbacks of the fall itself, when she is drifting off to sleep or in moments of quiet reverie, and relives the fall in stunning detail. About these flashbacks, she says: "I can feel the crash— actually feel how it felt at that moment when my head hit the roadway—and thinking 'Oh, crap, this is bad.'"

All during the winter, even though she is beginning to fill in some of the blanks, I detect in her a certain hesitancy when she talks about almost anything, as if she can't quite believe that she is getting back to her old self, getting back to normal. Her usual self-confidence has not returned fully. Many of her sentences are questions seeking affirmation from me as to the appropriateness of what she is saying, not declarations.

It's not, "The cognitive therapy sessions seem to be doing me some good" as much as it's, "The cognitive therapy sessions seem to be doing me some good?" her voice rising at the end in the suggestion of a question. She appears to be looking for confirmation that she is getting back to normal, a confirmation that can only come, in her mind, from the neurosurgeon pronouncing her—finally—sound, recovered, normal.

Ω Ω Ω

In early February, she has an appointment for another CT scan and, a few days later, an appointment with her neurosurgeon. Joanie wants, more than anything, to be normal: to be back to her old self, to be able to think and remember and speak as she did before sustaining that brain injury. But that injury has knocked so much of the self-confidence out of her, she is unable to judge for herself how normal she is. She accepts the family's assurances about how good she is doing and the progress we have noticed, but she accepts it with reservations. It will take only her neurosurgeon's pronouncing her normal for her to feel that she really is normal. Consequently, this followup appointment with Dr. Nanda looms, in her mind, as the most important hour she will spend in her life.

As I reflect upon it, I see why his pronouncement has such importance to her. Aside from the usual minor problems and challenges, both our lives have gone along at a good clip—happy childhood, good education, intense graduate study, a sound marriage, extraordinary children, satisfying jobs or volunteer work—all of it untainted by major illnesses, disappointments, or disasters. Now this. Joanie has so much to return to, to regain, but she can only get there by once again believing she is "normal."

And so we wait for the all-important meeting with her neurosurgeon. During the weekend intervening between the pre-appointment CT scan and the appointment itself, she tries to keep up a good front by going about her everyday affairs as usual, but her nervousness slips through. She tells me she worries that Dr. Nanda might see something untoward in her CT scan, that he might tell her there are problems inside her head, that he might restrict her from engaging in some activities. She tells me she worries most of all that he will *not* tell her she is back to normal. It is a long, anxiety-filled weekend for us both.

When the day of the appointment comes, the atmosphere around our house is as if we were leaving for a long trip, with all the attendant anxieties and concerns about our preparations for it and about whether or not everything will go well. We check and recheck the list of questions we had written out that we want to be sure Dr. Nanda addresses. I consult the, by now, thick file folder of information and notes about appointments, hospitals, and medications that have accumulated over the prior two months to make sure we have all our dates and facts straight. I even make sure that I've memorized Dr. Nanda's office number at Lahey so we can get to it as soon as we arrive at his building.

Joanie places herself in the safety spot in the center rear seat of the car, and I chauffeur her to Dr. Nanda's office at the Lahey Clinic. As we wait outside his office, our small talk with one another soon trails off into silence. There is nothing we can say to each other that would reach the import, in both our minds, that her neurosurgeon's words will.

Dr. Nanda comes into his examining room shortly after we are ushered into it. He calls up her latest CT scan on the screen right away. "That's a very normal brain," he pronounces. "It looks *very* nice." At that, Joanie's face lights up, but it takes a while for it all to sink in. Dr. Nanda shows us where, in earlier scans, blood from the hematoma can be seen and where, by contrast in the latest scan, none can be seen. He shows us where, in earlier scans, there had been fluid exerting pressure on her brain, and then in the latest scan there is none. He points out how her brain in the latest scan has returned to symmetry as opposed to the asymmetry caused by the considerable amount of fluid pressing on it that the earlier scans showed.

The visual evidence of the images seems to convince her: if it is there in black and white, it really must be true. It is what Joanie has been hoping for. No evidence of blood from her hematoma, her brain well-positioned within her skull—what Dr. Nanda considers "a normal brain." What her neurosurgeon has confirmed, she finally can acknowledge herself. She is back to normal.

The neurosurgeon does not recommend restrictions on her activity except, for three months afterward, anything that would cause bouncing or vibration to her head, such as jogging. He says there is no need for any further followup appointments with him.

At that, a wry smile coming over her face, Joanie quips, "You're a very nice man, Dr. Nanda, but I'm glad I don't ever have to see you again." We thank him for all he has done for us and leave.

Ω Ω Ω

Joanie continues with her cognitive therapy weekly for another three months as an outpatient at Emerson Hospital Outpatient Rehabilitation Center. These sessions illustrate that getting to complete recovery is going to be a marathon, not a sprint, a marathon run up peaks and down valleys.

With Mary Ann Butler, her outpatient therapist, she works primarily on her reading speed, spelling, memory for words, and word retrieval. Even into March, she still asks me how to spell words that, before her injury, she could spell easily. If she reads something aloud to me, she does it more haltingly and slowly than before. She tells me that sometimes when she looks at a word, it looks backwards to her. At other times, she is stymied by a word (usually a longish one), saying "I know what that word is, but I just can't say it." Words she doesn't use very often in everyday speech take a long time coming back to her.

It isn't just input, either; it's output, too. As she gets around to writing notes and e-mails again, she errs at times, substituting a wrong word for the correct one. In an e-mail to a friend several months after her accident, she writes, "I know you much be real busy." To another, she writes "Give my best to your did" rather than "dad." These were errors she would never have made before.

Her cognitive therapist has given her strategies to use when the processes she has used before don't work. One aid she suggests to assist her when reading aloud is to place an index card just below the line she is reading to help screen out other lines that might confuse her. Mary Ann also tells her not to interrupt her word search by expressing her frustration when she has difficulty coming up with a word she wants to use because that slows down her brain's momentum in its search for the word. Just keep using the strategies, Mary Ann urges her, and "you'll be more likely to get the word than if you give vent to your frustration at that moment."

After coming out from one of her cognitive therapy sessions with Mary Ann, Joan begins to tell me what went on. As we drive away from the parking lot of the rehabilitation facility, she suddenly interrupts herself by yelling out "colloquial!"

"What's that all about?" I ask.

"I just remembered it. Mary Ann had asked me to define some words that could have several different definitions. One of them was 'pop,' and one of my definitions was that it was a *something* word used for 'father'. You know, like Janna calls you 'Pop' sometimes. I couldn't remember what that *something* word was I was trying to use. I just now remembered; it's 'colloquial'."

A few weeks later, on our way to another session with Mary Ann, Joanie asks me if I have noticed any further improvement in her cognitive functioning.

"To tell you the truth, I haven't. Your reading is still very jumpy and hesitant and you're still having trouble finding words."

I don't relish telling Joanie that I haven't seen much progress over the last month that she had been working with Mary Ann, but since she asks, I feel she should have the benefit of my observation, especially since she is still seeing Mary Ann and will have a chance to work more on it in a concentrated, guided way.

Joanie says she will raise this at her next cognitive therapy session. After that session, when we are on our way home, she tells me what Mary Ann said.

"'Progress with this kind of injury to the brain is very slow,' Mary Ann told me. She said, 'Especially if your husband sees you every day, he's not going to notice much change from day to day. But look at how far you've come from two months ago.'"

And we agree that she is much better now, in late February, than she was in late December, right after her accident and surgery. "Mary Ann said that it could be a long time before I finish my recovery, but that I'll get there. We just have to be patient."

Ω Ω Ω

While the CT scan had shown her brain back in its normal position, several things still bother Joanie physically. Although her head pain is mostly gone, she still experiences fleeting pain over her left forehead where her stitches had been. At other times, she points out, it feels as if the pain were inside her scalp, below where the stitches were. She still has pain in her chest where a cracked rib was suspected. And one of her teeth doesn't feel right, causing her to wonder whether it may also have been injured in her fall against the asphalt that December morning. Her dentist later examines her and determines that there has been no permanent damage to her teeth. The other physical symptoms disappear very gradually with time.

Ω Ω Ω

After most of the rehabilitation therapists have discharged her, Joanie begins to pick up more of the strands that were a normal part of her life before the trauma to her brain happened. At the end of January, we meet Janna for dinner at a restaurant to celebrate my birthday, the first time Joanie and I have been out at night. One day a short time later, I leave her at home alone for most of the day while I go to an event a couple of hours' drive away.

We start going out together more around that time, mostly during the day, but a few times at night. One early February night, we go out to see the movie *The Queen*. Its star, Helen Mirren, is a favorite of Joanie's, and since the movie has already been playing for some time, she is afraid of missing it. She wears her cap to the theater, of course, but it gets so warm in the theater that she takes it off. After the movie, she slyly remarks that, even though the theater was dark, that still counts as the first time she's been in public without her cap.

Another evening, upon returning home after meeting some friends for dinner at a restaurant, Joanie gushes, "That was fun. It felt so normal. Since I don't have to take those medications anymore, I even had *two* glasses of wine with dinner . . . . It's so much fun to start to feel normal and do stuff we used to do."

In February, she begins to regain a level of comfort talking on the phone that she had lost in the prior two months. Much of her former vitality and sociability is returning. She is less chary about going out of the house on her own. She goes out to lunch with friends a couple of times in February. Around that time, she writes in an e-mail to one of her quilting pals:

> *I do feel like my brain is beginning to work as it should (except for my reading speed, spelling, and some memory). I also did the mystery quilt blocks cuz they were really easy to do—I'm not braggin —but it is nice to have something normal to do.*

Before her accident, she had started making a baby quilt when she had heard from our friends, Pat and Bert Hewitt, who were now living in Maryland, that they were going to be grandparents again. One day she picks it up and says, "The baby is getting to be a month old already. I better finish this quilt." And she does.

Next, she decides to make a quilted runner for our dining room table from a pattern her friend Ruth had given her some time before. As always when it comes to things for our house, she and I consult on colors and fabrics. Once we decide on them, Joanie finishes the piece in short order.

By the time March rolls around, she is well into doing a quilted hanging for five-year-old Hudson, another of Pat and Bert's grandchildren. We enjoy going to fabric stores together to pick out the novelty fabrics containing the cars, trucks, and dogs that we know Hudson likes, some of which are integrated into letters that she makes to spell out his name at the top of the hanging. Joanie and I have always had the same design sense and almost always agree on matters of design taste, whether in fabrics or furniture, so it is fun to look together for things for our house or for a quilt. Doing it now with her, after her accident, gives me assurance that things are returning to normal.

Ω Ω Ω

Although Dr. Nanda had pronounced her "normal" at her last appointment, and although we are now starting to resume "normal" activities, Joanie remains deliberate and cautious about certain things. Throughout all of February, whenever she has to go anywhere, I drive her. And if the drive is for any distance more than a couple of miles, she chooses to sit in the center of the back seat, the car's safest spot, rather than in front next to me. She wants to lessen the chances of even a minor accident injuring her head again.

Dr. Nanda had told her she could resume each of her normal activities as she felt comfortable to do each. She makes her first tentative moves to drive herself in March. In my car (which is a good nine years older than hers—she doesn't want to chance an accident happening to her newer car), we first take, with me beside her, small drives around the quiet streets of our neighborhood to make sure that she has the reflexes and strength to operate a vehicle. It is only in late April that she feels confident enough to resume driving her car completely on her own.

Throughout January, she continues to wear her Boston Red Sox cap whenever she is out in public, for her scar remains slightly visible under the wispy hair that has begun to grow over it. Not until mid-February has her hair grown long enough for her to feel comfortable being seen in public without the cap.

And for the longest time—not until March—does she wear shoes that have shoelaces.

Ω Ω Ω

When Valentine's Day comes around, Joanie demonstrates that she is recovering not only her mental functioning, but also her joy in life and her sense of humor. When I come downstairs in the morning, there is a Valentine card she had bought waiting for me. It is a humorous one showing a wife and husband sitting in their living room with dialogue bubbles emanating from the wife's head asking her husband questions women are stereotypically supposed to ask their sweethearts, such as "Does this make my butt look too fat?" and "Do you like these earrings on me?" The husband's bubbles answer, in turn, the one-word answers men stereotypically are supposed to give to those questions. On the card, Joanie had crossed out the woman's questions that were printed on it while leaving the man's printed answers unsullied. In place of the printed questions the woman on the card is asking, Joanie has written in the kind of questions that she has come to ask me repeatedly over the last two months. The "revised" card now reads:

Woman: Does my hair look weird?	*Man: No*
W: Is that spelled right?	*M: No*
W: Will I be dumb forever?	*M: No*
W: What's that word?	*M: No*
W: Want to go to Boston Bean?	*M: Yes*
W: Do I have to see Nanda again?	*M: No*
W: Do I need another CT scan?	*M: No*
W: Want to go for a walk?	*M: Yes*
W: Do you mind helping me exercise?	*M: No*

Ω Ω Ω

Although we continue to build her endurance for walking by taking short strolls together around the neighborhood several times a week, it is only in late February that she is able to make the three mile round trip from our house to Boston Bean and back. It comes about unplanned. Since Joanie's accident, I had also given up walking, and I was beginning to see the effects of that in the ten pounds I had gained during that time.

As I strode around our neighborhood with my wife to build up her endurance, I was also building up mine for my eventual return to walking. One morning, after a particularly unsettling meeting with my scale, I tell Joanie that I am going to walk to the Bean.

"Do you think I can do it with you?" she asks hesitantly.

"Sure, why not?"

I hadn't, until then, raised the idea of her resuming those three-mile walks, as I felt that when she was ready to, she would. On this day, we walk in triumph to Boston Bean House together for the first time in almost three months.

Three weeks later, on our third walk there together, we are sitting at our usual table, absorbed in our books. We don't notice our friend Linda run in to order a coffee, but as she runs out, coffee in hand, she detours to our table.

With a big grin on her face, Linda pronounces her benediction: "This looks right. This just looks right!"

By early March, I know that Joanie is ready to resume regular walks to the Bean when, about a mile out of our house on one of those walks, she begins to outpace me. The only thing holding her back from walking into Maynard completely by herself at this point is the snow and ice that had compacted from earlier snowfalls, making some of the spots on the sidewalks and the side of the road slippery. Fearing that another fall so soon after her accident would undo all her progress, we bide our time until the cold weather leaves, and with it the snow and ice that make the going iffy. April marks her first walk into Maynard by herself.

Spring

Even into the end of April, when her outpatient cognitive therapy sessions are winding down, Joanie still feels that not everything is quite right yet. In an e-mail to our son around that time, she writes:

> *Hi Darlin',*
>
> *My therapy has gone well, and I'm nearly back to my ol' self. I still have a little problem with word retrieval—I know what I want to say, sometimes I can even see the word in my mind, but I just can't get it out. My reading is also getting better, but it's still slower than it was and I still see a word that I don't recognize even though it's a word I know. All in all, however, I'm close enough to the way I was that only you guys (Dad and Janna, too) would know I'm not 100%. My speech therapist said that even after I finish with her (next Wed.), I'll continue to improve. I still do crosswords—the Sunday Globe and the two books Dad and I have that I was doing before. So, soon all this will just be an unpleasant memory . . . .*
>
> *Love, Mom*

Six months post-accident, she is still showing some hesitancy in her speech as she gropes for the right words, and she still has some reading problems. One day in early June, as we are sitting in Boston Bean House with our respective mystery novels, she remarks to me, "Sometimes I don't know how to pronounce a word I'm reading in a sentence, and so the sentence doesn't make any sense, and I have to go back and read the sentence three or four times. Finally, I realize it's a word I know how to pronounce and then the meaning of the sentence falls into place. Like in the Jonathan Kellerman book I'm reading, there are some psychiatric terms that look strange to me. But then I finally realize that I know those words—I just don't recognize them the first or second time I look at them." She describes further how, even at this point in her recovery, small words can throw her. "I see the word 'move' for example, and I say to myself 'voom?' That still happens at least once a day."

Ω Ω Ω

Around six months after her accident, after some short practice runs, we ride our bikes to Maynard for breakfast at the Boston Bean House. We park the bikes outside the shop so we can keep an eye on them through the window. As we sit reading at our usual table in the Bean, I notice out of the corner of my eye our friend Dorothy breeze in for a takeout coffee. She looks out the window at our bikes and then makes a special point of striding over to our table before she leaves.

She taps Joanie on the shoulder to get her to look up from her reading, then tells her, "I'm so inspired by how quickly you've gotten back on your bike."

"I feel I just had to, Dorothy. I don't want to be defined as the woman with the brain injury."

A few weeks after that, on Father's Day, a greeting card from Joan is waiting on the kitchen counter when I come downstairs in the morning. It is addressed to "My loving husband." Its printed message reads about how, in the face of life's unpredictability, her husband's love is always there for her.

This time, she didn't change a word that was printed on the card.

Summer

Throughout the summer and into the fall, Joan continues her recovery, getting stronger, building her confidence, and improving her speech and reading as each day passes. As summer rolls around, she resumes almost all her usual activities, which include visiting her mother at the nursing home, taking care of her mother's affairs, visiting her women friends on a more regular basis, resuming her quilting full bore, visiting Janna, keeping house, and, most of all, planning for the future.

We resume our usual activities as a couple, too, going out to dinner with friends, going in to Boston to see special exhibits at the Museum of Fine Arts, going to Red Sox games on those rare occasions when we can score tickets. As we get out more and run into some of our old friends and acquaintances who have not seen Joanie since before her accident, they ask her "How are you?" in a way that is subtly different from before. I hear a particular inflection in their question, which, to me, has the subtext of asking "Are you really back to normal, are all the pieces back in place, or are you permanently damaged in some way?" Whether Joanie notices it or not, the answer she gives to their question seems to reassure our friends that she is the same Joanie they previously knew. And they seem to be relieved not to have to walk on glass around her.

Janna calls us a few weeks before our fortieth anniversary on August 12 and tells us to hold open that date: she wants to have us over for dinner at her place to celebrate our anniversary. When that night comes, Joanie and I dress for our quiet dinner with Janna and leave for her place. When we get to her building, we ring her bell, she buzzes us in, we take the elevator to her floor, and we knock on her door. When she lets us in, we are met by a couple dozen of our friends yelling in unison "Surprise!"

Our daughter, who loves to cook up surprises for us, has done it again, big time this time. Neither Joanie nor I have the faintest idea that we are going to be doing anything other than spend a quiet evening with our daughter over dinner to celebrate our fortieth anniversary. The surprise party is a roaring success. We talk familiarly with our friends, have the food and wine Janna has laid out, and have a great time. It gives our friends the opportunity to see how well Joanie does in a big crowd, and it gives Joanie another confirmation that she is back to normal, back among the living.

Ω Ω Ω

Joanie decides that our twenty-seven-year-old house needs renovation and redecoration, and, after some initial resistance from me (after all, it appears good enough to me as it is), she manages to convince me that its single-pane windows, dark-stained woodwork, white walls, and red brick fireplace combine to make the house look dated. As a result, we plan the projects we think the house needs in order to update it, and we start on rounds of interviews with window replacement people, window treatment experts, painters, tilers, and other tradespeople as we try to decide what we should do and who to hire to do it. We then spend the following several weeks assessing the alternatives and trying to figure out how the changes might look and which of the options we are considering will fit into our budget. Once we make these decisions, there are long drawn-out rounds of deciding specifically which types of windows to purchase, what types and colors of window treatments to buy, what colors to paint the different rooms of our home and with what brand of paint, what types and colors of tiles to use on our fireplace, and on and on. The world has gotten a lot more complex and advanced since our house was built, and we haven't anticipated that there are so many different window technologies, kinds of window shades, colors and types of paint, and types of tile to choose from. But we make our decisions and schedule the work to be done during the fall, after we return from two much-needed vacations.

Each summer, one of my brothers, who lives in Switzerland, returns to the United States with his family for an annual home visit to see the rest of our family, using Maryland (where we grew up) as his base while in the States. When the time approaches for him and his family to come to the States, I ask Joanie, "Do you feel up to flying to Maryland to see the relatives when Charlie and Kiran and their kids are there?" I have a couple of motivations for asking her to go with me, beside the pleasure of her company. One is that each time she does something again after her accident that she has done before it, it confirms to her that she is getting better. She has not flown since before the accident, and I believe that flying once again would be another getting-back-on-the-bike experience for her.

My other motivation is that when I've talked on the phone with my siblings (none of whom live in Massachusetts), and they've asked how Joanie is doing, I can detect in their voice the same unasked questions our friends ask: "How's her health and her mind? Is she getting back to normal?" I want them to see for themselves that this is the same Joanie they knew before the accident and that she is recovering from her traumatic brain injury. I want them to see for themselves that she is no longer "the woman with the brain injury."

"Sure, if you want to see your family, I'll go," she says to me. And we do, flying from Massachusetts to Maryland and spending a long weekend there visiting my family as well as our long-time friends, the Hewitts. I can see that Joanie takes the experience in her stride, and that my family and our friends are relieved to see that Joanie is no longer "the woman with the brain injury."

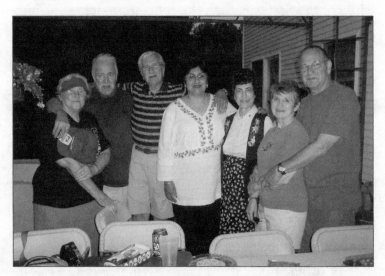

In Baltimore with (most of) the Kerpelman clan.

Ω Ω Ω

The flight to Baltimore is a practice run for a longer flight we take a month later. Several weeks before our fortieth wedding anniversary in August, I suggested that we go all out to celebrate it—and Joanie's recovery—with a cruise on the Baltic Sea. For a long time, ever since she had heard from friends how enchanting it was, Joanie had wanted to take a Baltic cruise. What better way to celebrate our fortieth than finally to do it (adding on a side trip to Switzerland after the cruise to visit my brother and his family there)?

Of course, we discuss whether or not Joanie both feels, and actually is, well enough to take the three-week-long trip. "What if I have a problem while we're on the boat or in one of the countries, 4,000 miles from home?" she wonders. We thoroughly discuss the possibilities and contingencies and, in the end, decide that her recovery is going so well that there is little chance of her regressing on that front. Besides, we both are convinced that health care in most of the countries the cruise will visit is at least on a par with that in the U.S., if not better. There is little reason not to go, we tell each other.

Consequently, throughout the summer we plan the trip and, in late August, fly to Copenhagen to embark on the cruise. Each port of call—Copenhagen, Stockholm, St. Petersburg, Tallinn, Gdansk, Oslo—is a real delight. On her birthday in September, the ship is in port in Tallinn, Estonia, a surprisingly delightful city with a medieval city center. Joanie is thrilled with being in a place as charming as Tallinn for her birthday. And in fact, she is thrilled with the whole trip, as am I. Nothing goes awry, there are no concerns on either of our parts about her health, and we so enjoy stepping back into life slightly outside our comfort zone.

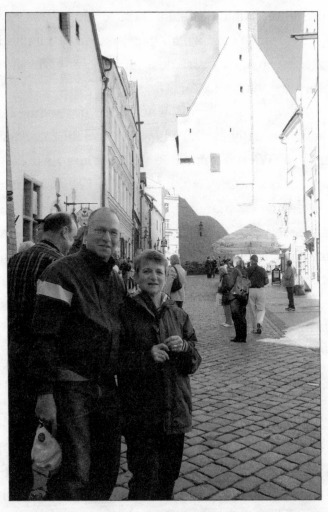

We celebrate Joanie's birthday in Tallinn, Estonia.

Autumn

Having made all the decisions before we left for Europe about which tradespeople to hire to do the updating of our house, and what materials would go into it, the work is ready to begin almost as soon as we return from the cruise. For most of the autumn, we have a constant stream of workers in our house as they move the look of our house from the twentieth into the twenty-first century. All of this Joanie handles with aplomb and her usual patience and grace, no small feat given that there are a corps of strangers—window replacers, painters, tile layers—virtually living in our house for days at a time as the work is being done. Joanie's mastery of the complexities and decisions involved in the entire project demonstrates that her mental competence and agility have returned. And having the house redecorated gives us both a sense of renewal, a concrete demonstration that the accident and all it has wrought is behind us.

Ω Ω Ω

Joanie graduates to feeling comfortable walking in to Maynard by herself on a regular basis—getting back her daily "zen moments." She is, to be sure, more cautious than she was before her accident, always making certain before she leaves the house that she has her cell phone with her. In fact, she tells me, "I now regularly think, more than I ever did before the accident, about where you are and where Janna is in case something should happen to me."

One day, she gathers all her shoes, and we determine which ones have laces that are too long for safety and which ones can pass muster on the lace-length score. She then has me cut down the laces that are too long. She insists that I do the same with my shoes.

She no longer carries the laundry basket up and down the stairs to and from our laundry room because, between its weight and bulkiness, it makes negotiating the stairs dangerous for her. She leaves it instead for me to take, and if I'm not around when it's time to take the basket down so she can do the laundry, the laundry waits. She is careful to leave a night light on overnight to lessen the possibility of tripping and falling in case she gets up at night.

"I still worry about myself more than I ever did before," she says one day. "And about other people who have suffered a brain injury, too. When Bob Woodruff [the television news correspondent] suffered that brain injury when he was in Iraq, seeing the reports on television about what was happening to him and the challenges he faced brought it all back again to me, even though his injury was so much worse than mine. I'm thankful that mine wasn't that bad, but I'm still angry that it happened to me at all.

"And I think a lot," she continues, "about how hard this all must have been on you and Janna and Todd. I didn't realize it at the time, when I was just trying to get back to normal, but I realize now all you guys did and how you must have worried."

I assure her we will always be there for her. It is good to have her back.

Ω Ω Ω

If you look at Joan closely now, you can see a slight dime-sized depression in her skin just above her left eyebrow. That piece missing from her skull is about the only piece of her physical being now missing. It will remain missing throughout the rest of her life as a reminder of the burr hole the neurosurgeon drilled through the dull ivory of her skull that stopped just at the outer lining of her brain.

8

ANNIVERSARY

IT HAS BEEN QUITE a journey for Joanie and me, the most trying, strangest journey of our forty years together. It has brought changes to our lives, but oddly, as many good ones as bad. We are both more cautious and careful about ourselves, our health, and our safety than we were before. We both look out for one another more conscientiously than we did before. We both count ourselves fortunate to have the caring friends and family that we have. We always had an appreciation of how fragile life is, but now we both feel it in our very cores rather than just understand it in our heads.

We are angry and saddened that Joanie had to endure this injury and undergo so much suffering, yet we are glad that she is now almost back to where she was before on both the happiness and the health fronts. Our love for one another has deepened beyond what we ever could have imagined before.

Her terrible injury brought our family even closer together. Both as a unit and individually, we helped Joanie heal and that, in turn, strengthened our family bonds. As soon as her mother was injured, Janna shuffled her teaching and living arrangements so she could be with her every possible minute. At some cost to her, she had other teachers take over her job responsibilities, and she essentially moved back to our house during this ordeal to be that much closer to her mother. There's no exaggerating the strength of the bond that she and Joanie have, and Janna's being there for her mother throughout the unfolding chain of events gave Joanie strength and courage.

Todd rearranged his work and home life to be with his mother at the most critical juncture of her recovery. He was supposed to be 3,000 miles away on the West Coast with his new wife and her parents that Christmas, and, instead, he set out to be with Joanie as she was recovering. He would have been with us sooner had I not kept dissuading him from flying in to be at his mother's bedside. Once he did come, his presence, his air of calm laced with humor, and his resourcefulness brought a sense of normality to our household. Especially having him home with Joanie, Janna, and me as Joanie began her recovery made a difference in that recovery. And being with us at Christmas made that Christmas seem much like Christmases past.

Between the daily, day-long visits to Joanie at the hospital and being with her at home after her hospital stays were done with, with Janna's help I was able to keep the wheels of our household moving, pay bills, see that shopping got done, and keep our friends and family informed of Joanie's progress. I served as her advocate, when an advocate was needed, to get the best of medical care and rehabilitation planning for her that I could. And I served as her "brake" to keep her from impeding her recovery by doing too much too soon.

During the year of Joanie's injury and recovery, people would often ask me how I was coping. I cannot really answer that I coped well or didn't cope well— maybe I did both. I was worried and harried facing my wife's pain, her hospitalizations, the many medical and rehabilitation visits, and her neurosurgery. But I benefited from having a circle of support among family and friends, good health, time to do all that needed doing, good health insurance coverage for Joanie, a basic (if rusty) understanding to start with of traumatic brain injury (which I supplemented once her injury happened), and the example of Joanie's determination and grit in recovering her lost capabilities to inspire me. Even my writing of the frequent e-mails to apprise our family and friends of Joanie's condition and progress provided me with a cathartic outlet.

I had learned from one of my closest supervisors during my working career the value of putting one foot in front of the other, no matter what came before or during, adopting his policy of "deal with it, but don't dwell on it—just keep on stepping" through adversity and obstacles. It wasn't easy for me to keep on stepping the year of Joanie's recovery, but it wasn't hard, either, when, as I often did during that time, I compared my travails with the pain and suffering Joanie was going through.

Joanie's contributions to her own recovery were instrumental in its going as rapidly and as well as it did. Once she had come out of her fog enough to realize what the accident had done to her, she showed courage, determination, and immense strength and stamina in getting back on her feet—figuratively and literally—as soon as she could. She didn't just do the ten reps of each exercise that the physical therapist instructed her to do—she did fifteen. She didn't just practice her reading exercises the day before her cognitive therapy appointments, she threw herself into them as soon as her therapist assigned them to her. Even a year after the accident, she kept up her strength and balance exercises to ensure that she would be in better shape than she was before it. She is ever so much more careful now to avoid potential accident-causing situations.

How did all this impact our relationship? Like most long-married couples, we had grown, over our four decades together, "old shoe" comfortable with one another and therefore a little complacent about expressing how we felt about one another. This accident changed all that. It made us feel in our hearts the things that we knew in our heads: about how fragile life is and how priceless our relationship with each other is. This accident taught me in a way nothing else could how bereft and empty I would be if I were to lose her, and it demonstrated concretely to her that our children and I would be there for her no matter what, to help her through whatever adversities she might face. Now, we value our time together with an intensity we had not felt for a long time. When Joanie goes upstairs to bed each night (before I do, as she's always done), it's never without a warm goodnight hug and kiss. Every day is a new and separate joy.

Ω Ω Ω

In many ways, Joanie had been holding her breath as we approached the one year anniversary of her accident. She was thinking that if she passed that milestone in her journey of recovery as a now-normal human being, she would be able to consider herself 100 percent whole, 100 percent cured, 100 percent her old self.

In that year, she had come a long, long way. Her verve, humor, and intelligence returned in full force. She had her life back, completely, our children had their mother back, and I had my wife back. Her reading, speech, and strength all returned to about where they were before her accident. For the most part, so had her memory. All except her memory of the period from December 8 to December 18. That has only come back very gradually, and I suspect that she will never fully know what happened to her during that time of such intense pain and suffering. Other than that piece missing from her past, and the slight depression on her temple, there are no more major pieces missing.

Ω Ω Ω

The week before the one-year anniversary of her accident, Janna and I plotted a small surprise for Joanie to mark that high point. I surreptitiously made reservations for dinner for the three of us at one of the more atmospheric restaurants nearby. Janna was to drive out from her home and meet us there. When Saturday of that weekend rolled around, I begged off going out to dinner with Joanie to the local Not Your Average Joe's restaurant (as had been our Saturday custom), telling her I was too tired. "But let's plan to go to Joe's tomorrow," I said ("tomorrow" being one year to the day of her accident).

Sunday evening we got into the car for our delayed night out. As we reached, and then drove past, Not Your Average Joe's, Joanie gave me a pointed, quizzical look.

"We're going somewhere else," I said with as much mystery as I could muster, and I continued to drive on.

When we arrived at the 5 Strawberry Hill restaurant, the plot was revealed. Janna was waiting for us there, having driven out from her place. We sat down to enjoy dinner, and, after the waitress poured the wine Janna had ordered for us beforehand, I proposed a toast.

"We're here to celebrate Mom's first anniversary of being past her accident," I announced, "but this will also be the last time we'll celebrate it. As Mom has said before, she doesn't want to be known as the woman with the brain injury."

After the toast, I gave Joanie an "anniversary gift" of two Boston Bean House jerseys. Janna gave Joanie a card and a gift—a *Life is good*® jersey. How appropriate, I thought. To my surprise, she gave me a *Life is good*® shirt, too, a gift, she said, to recognize how stressful the year had been for me as well, and in appreciation of what I had done to help her mother get her life back on track.

Ω Ω Ω

I sat alone later that night in the quiet of our family room, after Janna had driven back to her place and Joanie had gone upstairs to bed, reflecting on the year we had just celebrated and now put behind us. With tremendous fortitude and grace, Joanie had lifted herself out of the abyss of a traumatic brain injury and pulled herself back to the heights of living as she had before.

Our family—Janna, Todd, his wife Brooke, and I—had pulled together during the crisis to do whatever we could to help her get there. Our extended family, neighbors, and friends had all pitched in to provide us support—whether in the form of food, flowers, cards, visits, or just being there for us. The medical and rehabilitation people had done their jobs well.

As I was thinking about all this, my mind drifted back to something that occurred about two months earlier. That day, October 13, was another crystal clear, beautifully sunny day, almost a clone of that beautiful yet terrible Saturday the year before when Joanie fell and our lives changed. On that recent October day, as on the day the accident occurred, Joanie and I were walking into Maynard to have breakfast at the Bean.

As we walked, she asked me if I happened to see a segment earlier that week on one of the national morning television shows. "In that segment," she told me, "people were asked to summarize their life, or where they were at that moment in their life, in just three words and to write those words on their hand."

"No, I hadn't seen it."

Joanie introduced it to me by commenting how deeply emotional it was for her. "It showed people expressing highly charged sentiments, like 'Miss my soldier' and 'I love life.'

"The one that sticks in my mind was . . . ," but she couldn't finish her sentence. Her eyes welling up, she said, "I don't know if I can get this out."

We fell into a long silence and continued to walk as she tried to regain her composure. After several minutes, she took a deep breath and began to tell me about it. As she did, there were no resounding cheers, no triumphant fanfares. Only quiet tears of victory.

"The one I want to tell you about was the person who needed two hands to write her story.

"On the one hand, it said, 'I FELL DOWN.' On the other hand, it said, 'I GOT UP.'"

AFTERWORD

⁘

I DIDN'T DELIBERATELY plan to write this book;
obviously, I wish the accident that started it all and
triggered the events in the year that followed had not
happened at all. Seeing a spouse lying inert, in pain,
unable to recall things that happened to her, and
having difficulty finding words to express herself had
a way of concentrating my mind that was both intense
and personal. And it's that intense and personal feeling
that compelled me to write this book.

As I reflect back on the whole ordeal, I realize that
Joanie and I were so much more fortunate than many
people. Bad as it was, the situation could have been
worse—much worse. Joan had, after all, suffered an
injury beneath the outermost lining of her brain, not
within her brain itself. With a more severe injury, she
might have had a longer hospitalization, a different
and possibly more radical neurosurgery, and a longer
rehabilitation period. She could have suffered permanent
and pervasive brain damage, never returning to her
former level of either physical or cognitive functioning.
She could have died.

This is not to say that her brush with traumatic brain injury was smooth sailing. Joanie did suffer in one way or another most of the immediate effects almost all traumatic brain injury sufferers experience: extreme head pain, confusion, lethargy, nausea, sleep disturbances, impaired attention, memory loss, and emotional, behavioral, speech, and hearing problems. Seizures also often occur in traumatic brain injury victims, although that was averted in her case through the use of anti-seizure medication as a preventative. But the long-term effects of her brain injury on her were minimal.

Her recovery undoubtedly occurred faster than it otherwise might have because of her life style. Before the accident, she had kept herself in good condition physically, exercising daily and making certain that what she ate was healthful. Aiding her recovery was a strong support system of concerned and caring family and friends. I had retired from my thirty-year consulting career and could spend all the time necessary to be with her while she was in the hospital and afterward while she was at home recovering. Our daughter lived not that far away from us and could rearrange her working schedule (albeit with difficulty) to do the same. Our son flew in from California at an important juncture on Joan's road to recovery while his wife held down the fort at their home. Joanie manifested a rock-solid determination to return to health and, once the neurosurgery was behind her, threw herself into the rehabilitation exercises she was prescribed with a level of pure grit that was impressive to behold. She received good medical, surgical, nursing, and rehabilitative care. She had good health insurance that covered almost all the expenses we incurred in connection with her injury, and it did so almost seamlessly.

I cannot help but marvel at how people who suffer a traumatic brain injury, but who are not as fortunate to have all these things going for them, cope. This crisis gave me a better appreciation than I had before for those who have to deal with brain injury, both the sufferers and their families. It also gave me a better appreciation than I had before of the adaptiveness and plasticity of the human brain, an adaptiveness and plasticity that neuroscientists have been exploring progressively more fruitfully over the last several decades. When her head hit the roadway and began to bleed and swell, neurons were destroyed and pushed out of position, yet others eventually took over their functions.

My focus, and that of my daughter, son, and daughter-in-law were all inward on our family during the year of Joanie's injury, pain, hospitalization, surgery, and rehabilitation. Making the right decisions about Joanie, helping her recover, putting the pieces back together again dominated our lives that year.

As well as this experience ended for Joanie and our family, it also raised some nagging questions and concerns. I don't pretend to have all the answers to them, yet they are important to bring up just the same. Joanie's accident thrust me back into two areas I was familiar with through my career. Both my undergraduate and graduate educations had been in the field of clinical psychology. I didn't specialize in brain injury, but I did study it in the course of my graduate work, and very early in my professional career I had done clinical work, occasionally seeing patients with varying levels of brain damage. Still, there was so much more that I didn't know or remember about brain injury that I was to find out once my wife's accident occurred.

My subsequent career took me into the field of public policy research and consulting, where I managed projects in a variety of fields, a major one being health care. While not a out-and-out expert in that field (my expertise lay in research methodology that could be applied to any number of public policy fields, not in any one substantive field), through my professional career I gained a better than average familiarity with the American health care system. The accident, though, threw Joanie and me into a much more intimate, consumer's acquaintance with that health care system than either of us had before, or would care to have for that matter. That consumer's perspective gave me a far better idea than my academic acquaintance with the health care system ever could of both its high notes and low ones.

It's these topics—the U.S. health care system and traumatic brain injury—that I turn to here.

Health Care System

The United States has some of the best medical technology, research, and practitioners in the world, but that technology and research, and those practitioners, operate within a fragmented and incoherent health care and health finance system. It is a system that William Brody, recently president of The Johns Hopkins University and himself a physician, characterized as the industrial world's most inefficient medical system.

Brody echoed the collective opinion of the American College of Physicians, which, in a 2008 paper examining how to improve health care in the United States, pointed out the sad state of our system. Compared with commonly accepted benchmarks of health care quality in similar industrialized nations (such as the Netherlands, Belgium, and Canada)—and despite spending a larger share of its Gross Domestic Product on health care than any other nation in the world—the United States, according to this American College of Physicians study, falls short on a number of scores. These include poor coordination of health care services; a shortage of primary care physicians; wide variation in the cost, quality, and utilization of health care services; low usage of electronic medical record systems; disparities in health care access and delivery related to race, ethnicity, and socioeconomic status; and ineffective control (and therefore inefficient usage) of health technology.

The reasons for these shortcomings of the American system are many and complex. A tangled web of history, legislation, and regulation over the past half century, combined with the increased influence of health insurers and medical malpractice litigation on medical practice and health care provision—tossed up with a hefty portion of self-interest on the part of all the system's players—have all contributed to how that system has evolved and how health care in the U.S. is now provided. The health care and health insurance reforms debated and passed by the Congress during the Obama administration demonstrated how complex the problems are. And the resulting legislation demonstrated how incomplete those reforms could be in addressing them.

The individuals who are providing care within the U.S. health care system are, on the whole, well-trained, motivated, skilled, and caring, but the system in which they provide that care is disjointed and, as Brody indicated, inefficient. How much better health care provision in the U.S. would be if our extremely well-trained health care providers and our excellent technology could be allowed to work together in a more coherent way.

Looking at the U.S. health care system from a customer satisfaction viewpoint (a viewpoint that began to be powerfully applied in business near the end of the twentieth century) leads to the conclusion that the system still needs substantial change if the patients using it are to be served well. Applying some of those same customer satisfaction principles can help address those problems, in my opinion. While there is some movement of hospitals and health care providers toward being more truly consumer-oriented, there is still a way to go, particularly in the following areas.

Continuity of care. With the rise of the hospitalist phenomenon, primary care physicians often now assume the role of passive receivers of information about the hospitalized patients for whom they normally have primary concern. Joanie had at least three different hospitalists caring for her during her first hospital stay of four days. Her primary care physician did not see her during that time, nor during her second hospitalization, either (she changed her primary care physician shortly after her second hospitalization, partly as a result of this).

A 1998 article in *Physicians News Digest* states: "About 2000 physicians nationwide call themselves hospitalists. Specializing in the management of hospitalized patients, the hospital becomes their office. A hospitalist takes over for a primary care physician when it comes time to admit a patient. For your average primary care physician, this means fewer, or no, visits to the hospital at the end of their office hours for rounds. Usually working on flexible, yet intense shifts of eight to twelve hours, the hospitalist turns his or her pager off when the shift is over."

In just eight short years after that article was published, the number of hospitalists practicing in the U.S. was estimated to have grown to 12,000, with the expectation that it will eventually grow to 30,000.

Since a key role of the primary care physician is to manage health care for the whole patient, turning that care over to hospitalists while the patient is in the hospital (even if the hospitalists keep the primary care physician apprised) weakens that key component of caring for the whole patient. Moreover, a hospitalist does not have the same sense of connection with a patient that the patient's primary care physician has. Plus, since different hospitalists often see the patient during a hospital stay, there is a greater chance that communication about each case is, perforce, going to be less clear than if only one person, the primary care physician, is handling the case.

Those in favor of the hospitalist movement counter that the hospitalist, being based in the hospital, is more available to both the patient and the nurses who provide care for the patient than a primary care physician, whose office is often not in or near the hospital, would be. Should untoward developments in a patient occur, the hospitalists are there to act. In addition, because they work defined shifts, hospitalists tend to be fresher and more alert than primary care physicians, who may see their hospitalized patients at the middle or end of a busy day, would be. Those sympathetic to the hospitalist movement also point out that hospitalists' treatment and activities are monitored more closely by the hospitals in which they work than are those of primary care physicians providing care to their hospitalized patients.

All things considered, though, it seems to me that the major benefit of having a hospitalist care for a hospitalized patient accrues mainly to the primary care physician, who no longer has to suffer the inconvenience and wear and tear of visiting the hospital to see his or her patients, nor suffer the inadequate reimbursement that insurance companies provide for such visits. It's the patient who gets the short end of the stick in terms of continuity of care, in my opinion. Although she is seen by hospitalists while in the hospital, she is not necessarily seen by the same one during the course of her stay, potentially leading to communication disconnections among providers and disruptions in continuity of care. Even if the patient is seen by the same hospitalist throughout her hospitalization, she does not receive the benefit of being seen by a physician—namely, her primary care physician—who has an in-depth understanding of her, her prior history, and her health concerns.

The point that some raise, that hospitalists' treatment and activities are monitored more closely than are those of primary care physicians seeing their hospitalized patients, is hardly relevant. It implies that primary care physicians cannot be monitored as closely, but what is to say that they cannot? They may not be *used to* being monitored so closely, but that does not mean that they *cannot* be. Changes in hospital practice happen all the time (albeit slowly).

The medical community itself is not unaware of these issues, as they are a matter of vigorous discussion in the medical literature. An acquaintance of mine, an internal medicine physician who very much favors the hospitalist system, recognizes that most patients do not agree with him. "Patients hate it," he plainly admits.

Although the whole hospitalist issue is still a work in progress in the medical community as it tries to adapt to this change and perfect its workings, I think that the medical community is inclined to believe that the tradeoffs are worth it to them. From the health care consumer's point of view, however, the tradeoffs are not. Perhaps the vigorous discussion in the literature will come to encompass an examination of the shortcomings I have pointed out here and result in the provision of hospital care that is more satisfying and continuous.

Yes, one of the kindest, most caring individuals who saw Joanie during her first hospitalization is a hospitalist. But it was principally Dr. Halporn's dedication to his patient, not the fact that he is a hospitalist, that resulted, in Joanie receiving just the kind of care and treatment she needed during her crisis. As good as Dr. Halporn was in that situation, he was working within a fragmented system. It was only because he took it upon himself to break out of the role of being a cog in that system and into the role of being a health care case manager that he was able to provide the kind of continuity of care and case management that Joanie needed at a critically important moment, the moment when I found her in bed unresponsive and barely conscious after her first hospitalization. We were so fortunate that he was thoughtful enough to give me his cell phone number and so was there to guide me through that critical incident.

Even in the other hospital (Lahey Clinic) where she was not cared for by hospitalists, it was hard to figure out who had the big picture when it came to the total patient. The nurses were often helpful and informed about Joanie's day-to-day condition, but the questions we had of more long-term import, or those that concerned specific medical details, were always referred to the physicians for answers. As a result, we had to withstand long delays before we received answers to important questions we had. And even then, we got the feeling that the physicians were more concerned about her physical recovery (as important as that was) than her cognitive recovery.

We relied on her neurosurgeon and his associates when they were around, but I didn't have the impression that there was one person who had an *overall* view of the *entire* patient, not just her medical condition. I consider it illustrative that it wasn't until the next-to-last day of her ten-day stay at the Lahey Clinic hospital that someone who introduced herself as my wife's case manager appeared on the scene. Perhaps she was working behind the scenes all along, but it sure would have allayed a lot of anxiety within our family to have known that she was a resource we could have turned to right from the beginning, not the day before her discharge. (A social worker did visit us early in Joanie's stay at Lahey, but she left me with the impression that she served as an ombudsman, not a case manager).

One writer, describing his "six-month journey into the maddening, spirit-killing bureaucratic crannies of the health care system" to obtain appropriate care for his mother, thought he finally found a solution to his problems in the case management system. But he, too, was disappointed when he found out that he had to traverse seemingly insurmountable obstacles to obtain such service. He concluded, regarding any health reform that might take place, "Nothing will change at the only level where it really matters—the patient—unless reforms address the single most basic necessity: having the left hand know what the right hand is doing."

A good part of the problem is that in the health care world, especially the hospital world, the patient is not really the main customer who has to be kept satisfied. To the hospital, patients are, in many ways, short-term stakeholders. Hospital administrators have to keep a number of longer-term constituents satisfied, for it is with them that the hospital's ability to function lies. Primary among these long-term constituents are their medical staff, whose referrals and cooperation keep the hospital running; regulators, whose regulations and requirements must be met if the hospital is to be certified to provide certain types of care; and insurers, who pay most of the bills and who, unfortunately, drive many of the medical decisions. Medical personnel, in turn, also have to worry about insurers, whose primary interest is in keeping costs down, and regulators, whose concerns about how health care is provided cause them to look over the shoulders of the health care providers— intrusively, many of the latter would say. Regulators and insurers, for their part, try to keep fraud and abuse from happening, often by drawing up rules and regulations that have the unintended consequence of discomfiting patients and second guessing health care providers. And medical personnel also have to worry about a lawyer bringing a malpractice suit on behalf of a patient if the outcome of a case is not perfect.

In this web of interlocking interactions, where is the patient? Way down near the bottom of the list of constituents that are considered, served, and satisfied. In most other organizational systems, the direct customer—the one who receives the direct services offered—is the focal point. Businesses strive hard to satisfy that customer because that is where their bread and butter lies. But in the business of health care, the patient is often the least direct customer, and so the patient's satisfaction is often of the least concern to the other actors in the system.

Communication. From a customer satisfaction standpoint, it does not add to a hospital patient's comfort level if the patient asks questions about his or her health and treatment and it takes hours to get answers. Often the questions reflect an anxiety on the part of the patient that a ready answer to the question might allay. Earlier, I wrote of several occasions when it took hours for us to get a reply to even the simplest of questions or requests. This is a result of the chain of command in the system, where the physician is the ultimate authority. An answer to a question has to wait until a question asked by a patient or a family member gets to the physician through an intermediary (usually a nurse or a patient care technician), the physician provides an answer in some form, then the answer or decision trickles down to the nurse or patient care technician, who, finally, gives it to the patient or her family—hours or even days later. Within that chain, there is also the distinct possibility that the

communication will get garbled on its way up from, and
back to, the patient. No doubt this system has evolved
in order to avoid having incorrect or contradictory
information filter down to the patient. But does *every*
inquiry from a patient have to be handled this way? Is
there not some way to make the system more efficient
and therefore more effective?

Surely, with modern information technology
systems, this cumbersome question-response chain
doesn't have to happen. Businesses have learned that
they have to make their customers' experience with
them as pleasant and convenient as possible if they
are to be looked upon favorably by their customers,
which means, in part, providing error-free chains of
communication and swift and consistent answers to
appropriate questions from their customers. Health
care systems (especially hospitals) haven't learned
how to do that yet. I am not even sure they are aware
that it is a matter of concern and frustration for their
consumer-patients. Hospitals have, in many ways, a
captive audience, so perhaps they don't feel the need
to be highly responsive to their patients. Yet there is no
reason to put the patient constituency at the bottom of
the information pyramid.

I know it doesn't have to be so, for I have the example
of the Emerson Hospital Home Care organization to
look to. It was clear from the outset of our dealings with
them that the half dozen or so providers of outpatient

rehabilitation services from that organization (which in itself is a sub-unit within the larger Emerson Hospital) who saw Joanie knew her medical history, the details of how her accident occurred, and what was going on with her day-to-day during her rehabilitation. It was also clear that all the rehabilitation therapists who worked with her shared their information about her with one another and so could address without delay most of the questions we raised. I commented to one of the rehabilitation therapists how remarkable this seemed to me, given our experience with the hospitals, and I asked her how this was so. I expected her to tell me that they shared a common database that they could access on the laptop computers they all carried, and perhaps that was, indeed, a major factor in their ability to communicate smoothly and efficiently among themselves and with us. But the answer she gave me was a lot simpler: "We talk to one another." Granted, her organization is a much smaller and less complex one than the hospital as a whole, but it demonstrates that good communication isn't an insurmountable goal for a health care organization to reach.

Here again, I think that a fully realized and properly functioning case management system would help immeasurably in speeding communications and clearing the air of problems and misunderstandings. If there were a case manager whose focus is primarily to serve the patient and his or her family, ensure that the information flow between and among hospital staff and patient is clear and uncluttered, and keep them all informed, the kind of communication problems and delays I describe here would be minimized.

I have mentioned several times in this book the fact that Joanie was asked the same questions repeatedly about her past medical history and her recent accident. Some of the reason for this repetition is to make sure all the details come out, just as the police ask suspects and witnesses, over and over, to tell them what happened in the hope of turning up new information each time. It wasn't, for example, until about the fourth time Joanie recounted her accident (when telling our daughter in the hospital about her fall—that she caught her foot in the extra-long bow that her extra-long shoe laces necessitated) that the exact details of how she was pitched forward onto the road surface came out. The health care workers never know what information patients will say to whom, and knowing the mechanism of how an injury occurred is important.

A nurse friend tells me that nurses are required to draw up their own care plans and notes, and they must do this with information obtained directly from the patient. She also tells me that often they also do this to check the neurological status and the limits of a patient's recall and memory.

Joanie's answers to the repeated questions asked her were duly recorded most of the time. But I had the impression that those records were not shared fully across people, disciplines, or units within the hospital, and that some of the health care providers who asked these questions didn't bother to look to see if they previously were asked of, and answered by, the patient. I doubt it was laziness on their part; rather, I suspect it was because this information, while available, was just not that accessible. More widespread use of computerized medical record keeping would go a long way toward making patient information more accessible to health care providers.

From a customer satisfaction standpoint, it doesn't instill confidence in a patient that one of her health care providers asks her the same questions that another one had asked just a few hours or days before (usually without any explanation for the repetitive questioning). What it does instill in patients is exasperation with the system that is subjecting them to it and a nagging concern that one health care provider may not be passing on information to other providers.

Peace and quiet. I always had thought that hospitals were places where patients could receive rest to help them recuperate. Being with Joanie in the hospital every day gave me the impression, however, that keeping noise down was not a large consideration, at least among some health care providers we encountered. The jangling of hospital carts as they are pushed along hard floor surfaces, the ringing of telephones outside of hospital rooms, the conversations of the staff at nurses' stations all add up, noise-wise. When I mentioned to one of Joanie's nurses at Emerson Hospital how surprisingly noisy I found that place to be, she assumed a defensive posture, telling me, in so many words, "We have our jobs to do here. You can't expect us to try to keep the noise down as well." As if quiet shouldn't be part of the hospital environment.

If this is typical of attitudes among hospital staff, then they need better training about reducing noise and the reasons to do so. And if the amount of mechanical clatter I found was at all typical, then hospital physical plants need to be better designed or altered to make a greater dent in reducing it.

Jo M. Solet, of Harvard Medical School, described the problem and its implications this way: "Noise in health care facilities has increased by multiples in past decades, and it has a negative effect on health in several ways . . . . [including] increased stress and disrupted sleep for patients, lost privacy, communication errors, and clinician burnout." Dr. Solet goes on to point out that the 2010 edition of *Guidelines for Design and Construction of Health Care Facilities* has taken an important step in recognizing the need to control hospital noise by establishing minimum acoustic standards.

It has been demonstrated in numerous locations that identifying noise sources, modifying equipment and procedures, and educating staff—all relatively straightforward and easy-to-implement procedures—can effect noticeable reductions in hospital noise levels and in turn improve patient and staff well-being. Some hospitals (for example, Johns Hopkins Hospital in Baltimore, Women's Hospital of Baton Rouge, Louisiana, St. Mary's Hospital in Rochester, Minnesota, and Massachusetts General Hospital in Boston) have been successful in reducing hospital noise levels through just such steps. These are one-off demonstrations showing that the problem can be attacked fruitfully. Maybe we shall be able to see more systematic, sustained progress on this front in the future.

A big offender with regard to not just privacy but also noise is the semi-private hospital room where only a thin curtain separates one bed, one patient, and one patient's health care providers from the person or persons on the other side of the curtain. In Joanie's semi-private room, we could hear what was going on on the other side of that curtain without even trying, or, for that matter, wanting to try. Granted, semi-private rooms are the norm in hospitals of a certain age, but that doesn't mean that some retrofitting cannot be done to cut down the noise, given advances in recent years in sound-deadening materials, noise-attenuating technologies, and the like. The 2006 edition of the above-mentioned *Guidelines for Design and Construction of Health Care Facilities* mandated that only private rooms be built in new health care facilities, but it will likely be many years before fully private rooms will be the norm in hospitals.

Again, if this were a business problem, it would have been solved by businesses more expeditiously and creatively with innovative design, construction, and retrofit solutions for the physical plant, procedural modifications within the organization, and staff training in noise reduction. Hospitals need to devote more attention to addressing this issue meaningfully.

Protection of privacy. The Health Insurance Portability and Accountability Act (HIPAA) of 1996 (Public Law 104-191) contains within it provisions for the protection and privacy of individually identifiable patient information. Under HIPAA, health care providers are required to maintain patient confidentiality and protect private health information. That is all well and good, and it has indeed resulted in great improvement in recent years in the protection of patient privacy in health care matters.

But all the best intentions and rules and regulations go out the window (or, more accurately, over to the other side of the curtain) when a patient is in a semi-private room. In that setting, if you are in one bed, the usual thin fabric curtain between beds provides a certain amount of visual privacy, in that the people on the other side cannot see what is going on, but not much sound privacy (or speech privacy, as it is termed by health care facility designers).

With just that thin curtain between the beds, speech privacy, and with it information privacy, are just about non-existent. Discussions of the most personal matters between health care providers and patients or between patients and their visitors are hardly private and confidential with solely a thin curtain to block that information from being heard elsewhere in the room. Just the fact that we heard virtually every word passing between Joanie's roommate, the roommate's physician, and her relatives when, in fact, none of them directed a single word toward us speaks volumes, as it were, about confidentiality of information—a lot of it very private information—in that kind of situation.

How can we have all these HIPAA rules and regulations about privacy and yet have such an evident flaw in the system? The 2006 guidelines for the design and construction of health care facilities recognize this flaw in calling for only private rooms in new construction. Another recently proffered solution is a sound-absorbing privacy curtain called the Hush Curtain™ that reduces noise and increases speech privacy in health care facilities that still have semi-private rooms. With many semi-private (or less than semi-private) hospital rooms still existing in U.S. hospitals, most of which are equipped with flimsy cloth "privacy" curtains separating the beds, it is unrealistic to expect that the speech privacy problem will disappear quickly. But it is not unreasonable to expect that more effort be expended in ameliorating the problem that exists now and will continue to exist for the immediate future.

In a country known for its innovation and ingenuity, other serious efforts need to be made to install more sound-attenuating curtain fabrics, or to examine the effectiveness of the type of folding screen that is found in places like hotel function rooms, or to develop electronic sound-deadening mechanisms to keep private conversations private. Again, business and industry has solved problems like this, and I am sure that with greater attention paid to it, the lack of speech privacy in hospitals can be addressed more effectively.

Health insurance. Glaring by its omission up to this point in this book is any extended discussion of health insurance. Certainly, the whole health care finance system in the United States is deserving of overhaul, as the medical establishment, politicians, newspapers and magazines, concerned citizens, and even films like Michael Moore's *Sicko* have all called for. The U.S. health insurance system is disjointed (as is our health care system itself), overly complex (as is our health care system), and not patient-friendly (again, just like our health care system). Recent health care reform legislation in the U.S. has addressed only some of these problems.

Based on our experience with Joanie's hospitalizations and recovery, I have pointed out what I see as inadequacies and problems in the American health care system. Yet I cannot describe or discuss any problems with health insurance *based on our experience*. The reason is that we had none.

When I retired from my job, and my group insurance through my employer stopped, I had Joan covered through a direct-pay individual Health Maintenance Organization plan with Blue Cross Blue Shield of Massachusetts. Is such a non-group, non-employer-based, non-government-funded insurance plan expensive? Yes it is, if you consider the over $7,000 per year in premiums for her coverage expensive. But all through the unfortunate events that transpired during the course of her several emergency room visits, hospitalizations, and subsequent rehabilitation therapies, her health insurance functioned seamlessly. We had no paperwork to fill out throughout all of these occurrences, we had few bills to pay except for relatively minor co-insurance or deductible payments, and, after providing our insurance information to each hospital (which in turn made it available to the medical providers who rendered services to Joanie), we experienced no hassles or even questions from these providers as to who would pay our bills and when. I did not have to get involved in making sure that this procedure or that hospitalization was covered by her insurance, nor did I have to be overly concerned that her insurance would not pay the bulk of the large hospital and medical bills that mounted up. With all the other problems we were facing, it was comforting in the extreme not to have this other, potentially large, issue looming over us.

For treatment and care that cost thousands and thousands of dollars (as I confirmed by reviewing the claims our insurer paid), our out-of pocket expenses (for the aforementioned co-insurance and deductible payments) were little more than one percent of the total sum. While the whole issue of health insurance in the United States is complex, and while many people have justifiably complained about the costs and coverage of health care insurance, my experience with the insurance coverage of my wife's treatment for her injury gives me no cause to criticize here.

Brain Injury

The injury to her brain that Joanie suffered drove me to find out more about traumatic brain injury (TBI) and how it is experienced by, and affects, its victims and those around them. I want to share that information so that others who have come to suffer from this devastating injury (and their families and friends) know what to expect, how to cope with it, and, with any luck, overcome it.

Joanie was one of close to 2,000,000 Americans who suffered a traumatic brain injury that year. The most

reliable government estimate of the incidence of TBI in
the U.S. presently is that 1.7 million cases of traumatic
brain injury occur annually. *That's one traumatic brain
injury every 18-1/2 seconds in the United States.* These
estimates are on the low side, moreover, for they do not
count people who suffered a traumatic brain injury but
did not seek care for it.

Of those individuals in the U.S. who sustain a TBI
each year, more than 1.3 million visit an emergency
department, 275,000 are hospitalized, and 52,000
die. Further, each year an estimated 80,000 to 90,000
Americans are permanently disabled as a result of these
injuries. The economic burden of TBI in one year in
the United States alone is estimated to be 60 billion
dollars. These statistics have led one expert in the field
(himself a victim of traumatic brain injury as a child)
to characterize the situation as a national epidemic
and several others, pointing to the lack of education
and public awareness of TBI, to characterize it as a
silent epidemic. Obviously, the traumatic brain injuries
experienced by military personnel in the wars in Iraq
and Afghanistan have added to this epidemic.

The highest rates of traumatic brain injuries in
the U.S. occur among children ages 4 years and under
(1,121 per 100,000 population), older adolescents ages
15 to 19 (814 per 100,000), and the elderly ages 75 and
over (659 per 100,000). In almost every age group, TBI
rates are higher for males than females. Falls are the

leading cause of TBI, with some 398,000 fall-related injuries (28% of all TBIs) occurring annually in the United States. The rates for falls are highest among those ages 4 and under (594 per 100,000) and those ages 75 and older (360 per 100,000). The other causes of traumatic brain injuries are, in this order, other or unknown causes (22%), motor vehicle and traffic causes (20%), "struck by or against" events (19%)—where the injury is caused by being struck by (or striking) an object or person, as might occur, for example, in sports injuries—and, lastly, assaults (11%). Although falls are the leading cause of TBI for both children and elderly adults, they are the more prevalent cause of TBI among the elderly, representing 51% of all causes among older adults against 39% of all causes among children. Motor vehicle–traffic is the second leading cause in these age groups, accounting for 11% of TBIs among children and 9% among older adults.

Traumatic brain injury can be mild, moderate, or severe. With mild injury, there is often little or no loss of consciousness. The injured person may suffer from headache, confusion, lightheadedness, dizziness, blurred vision, ringing in the ears, a bad taste in the mouth, fatigue or lethargy, changes in sleep patterns, behavior, or mood, and trouble with memory, concentration, attention, or thinking. A person with moderate or severe TBI may show any or all of these symptoms plus persistent headache, repeated vomiting, convulsions or seizures, inability to awaken from sleep, dilation of one or both pupils, slurred speech, weakness or numbness in the arms or legs, loss of coordination, and increased confusion, restlessness, or agitation. In the worst cases, the individual may go into a stupor (that is, may become unresponsive but may be aroused briefly by a strong stimulus), a coma (that is, may become unconscious and unaware of his or her surroundings), or a persistent vegetative state (that is, may remain in a coma-like condition for a month or more).

Although little can be done to reverse the *initial* brain damage caused by trauma, individuals suffering a traumatic brain injury should, nonetheless, seek medical attention as soon as possible. This is so medical personnel can try to stabilize the individual and prevent further injury. A patient with suspected traumatic brain injury is likely to be taken for imaging tests to help determine the diagnosis and prognosis. These can include skull and neck X-rays and CT scans.

About half of severely brain-injured patients will require surgery to remove or repair hematomas or contusions (bruised brain tissue). Surgery may reduce or relieve the various symptoms of TBI.

Preventing traumatic brain injury. All of these facts and statistics suggest that it is better to prevent a head injury than to treat one. They suggest, further, steps everyone should take to prevent traumatic brain injury to themselves and others.

"Most traumatic brain injuries shatter more than one life," William Winslade, one of the foremost writers in the field, has written.

For infants and young children, every effort should be made to prevent falls from heights. This means not letting children play on tables, putting up removable gates at stairways to keep children from falling down the stairs, and placing bars on windows, if necessary, to keep them from falling out. While window screens may appear to be sufficient to hold children in, they should not be relied upon to keep children from pushing through them.

As children get older, they should be taught to use helmets or appropriate head gear for various activities. If that is done, they will soon see it as a natural accompaniment to the sport or activity. Helmet use should be encouraged for such activities as bike riding, skating, skiing, snowboarding, and skateboarding. In organized sports, helmet use should be required at all times, not just in games but in practices, too. In a sport that does not typically call for headgear, soccer, there is evidence to suggest that heading the ball can be injurious to young brains, so its younger participants should be discouraged from heading the ball until such time as wearing helmets becomes a matter of course in that sport.

In all sports, in all ages, participants should be discouraged from "playing through" injuries, especially head injuries. Newspapers are full of stories of athletes—amateur as well as professional—who have done this, with the full encouragement of their coaches, trainers, even parents, only to suffer severe consequences. Baseball pitcher Matt Clement was hit on the head by a line drive in 2005 and returned to the mound less than two weeks later. His career took a nosedive afterward. Preliminary findings from a study conducted at the Boston University School of Medicine identified chronic traumatic encephalopathy in the brains of six football players who all died before the age of fifty. This progressive condition results from repeated head trauma and can bring on early dementia and depression. Professional wrestler Chris Nowinski received several concussions while playing college football at Harvard and during his professional wrestling career. He describes the resulting years of mental confusion and forgetfulness in his 2007 book *Head Games*. In that book, he also mentions three high school football players who died within months of one another after receiving blows to their heads during games.

This list of the injured is long and would be even longer if all the non-professional athletes who suffer head injuries and then "play through" them (to their detriment) were even known. The important points to remember are (1) don't ignore a head injury; rather, seek medical attention immediately, (2) don't "play through" a head injury, even if encouraged to do so by others, and (3) be aware that having a second head injury within a year of the first can bring on severe, sometimes life-threatening, complications, so take every precaution to avoid a second one, especially during that critical first year afterward.

With automobile-traffic accidents the largest category of known causes of traumatic brain injury, it makes absolutely no sense at all for anyone to ride in an automobile without using a seat belt (or, among younger children, without being strapped properly and securely into a car seat). Adult seat belt use goes hand-in-hand with child seat belt use. Nationwide observational research sponsored by the National Safety Council found that when the driver is buckled, restraint use for children (fifteen years and younger) in the car reaches 87%, but when the driver is not buckled, only 24% of children are restrained in their seats. In vehicles with air bags, seat belts, properly used, are still absolutely necessary to reduce the incidence and severity of head injury. Air bags are supplementary safety devices; by themselves, they are nowhere near as effective in preventing injuries as are airbags plus safety belts. Those who ride motorcycles should use helmets at all times. With no steel cage or air bags to protect them, the risk to motorcyclists of TBI is great when riding accidents occur.

The elderly are most subject to traumatic brain injury from falls. Weakness, problems with balance, diminution of coordination, and slowing down of reflexes all contribute to this. Consequently, a number of steps should be taken to lessen the chance that the elderly will suffer a fall and a consequent TBI. Recognition by those around them that this is the case will help, as this will lead them to offer assistance to older people in going up or down stairs, navigating level spaces, and so on. Hand rails should be installed where there may not be any (such as on porch steps) and kept in good condition once they are installed. Living spaces should be inspected for danger spots that may cause falls (such as raised thresholds, loose rugs, and slippery surfaces). Appropriate footwear should be worn by the elderly to further reduce the possibility of slipping and falling. Since the vision of the elderly is not as good as that of younger people, hallways should be well-lit for them. Hallways fifteen feet or more in length should have a light at each end. The elderly should use assistive devices—be they canes, walkers, or wheel chairs—whenever appropriate. Since the bathroom, with all its hard and slippery surfaces, is a particular danger spot, grab bars that meet the Americans with Disabilities Act guidelines for safety should be installed in showers, tubs, and bathroom walls.

With 11% of traumatic brain injuries resulting from assaults, the obvious advice is to try to avoid situations where assaults may occur. Of course, in most cases, one may not know where or when a situation could result in an assault. The one exception here is the case where the person is in an abusive relationship. The best advice in that case is to leave that relationship as quickly as possible, as if your life depends on it. It might. Physicians, health care centers, and community agencies can all help. There are numerous local support organizations that will help a person leave an abusive relationship, providing information on real-life practical steps to take before, during, and after the getting-out process and helping the abused person take those steps.

If traumatic brain injury occurs. Inevitably, though, despite all reasonable precautions, a head injury may occur, and if that happens, seek treatment immediately, either in a hospital emergency room or with a primary care physician. We almost didn't—after all, Joanie's fall appeared outwardly to have resulted only in lacerations and abrasions to her face, and we were inclined to "wait it out" and see what developed. Obviously, had she demonstrated persistent headache, nausea, confusion, or similar serious symptoms, we would eventually have gone to the emergency room, but we are so glad that our primary care physician's office recommended that we go to the emergency room immediately. Little did we know what was going on inside her head until the emergency room physician pronounced "Well, I know why you have such a bad headache. Your CT scan shows a subdural hematoma on the left side of your brain."

If you or someone you know is a victim of a traumatic brain injury, you or your family will want to seek out sources of information and support to help you cope with the situation after the immediate crisis is past. Fortunately, there are a number of sources aimed at helping patients and their families deal with the new and often baffling circumstances surrounding TBI. What follows is by no means a comprehensive list of resources, nor is inclusion in this list meant to imply an endorsement, but it is a good place to start.

A number of organizations focus on brain injury and its effects. Some, such as the Brain Trauma Foundation, www.braintrauma.org, and the North American Brain Injury Society, www.nabis.org, address primarily professionals and focus mainly on research and education aimed at advancing the state of knowledge and treatment of brain injury. The information on their Web sites, though, provides a useful place for the non-professional to obtain a further understanding of traumatic brain injury.

Other sources offer advocacy and support for victims of brain injury in addition to education and information about brain injury. The Brain Injury Association of America is arguably the largest and best known of these. It is a research, education, and advocacy organization that offers a number of practical resources for brain injury sufferers and their families. Its Web site (www.biusa.org) is probably the best place to start to investigate the resources available for someone with a brain injury. On it can be found facts about brain injury, descriptions of treatment and rehabilitation resources, a general discussion of medications used in treating brain injury, publications on the topic that are for sale at its on-line bookstore, and fact sheets on various aspects of brain injury. The Brain Injury Association has chartered state affiliates in forty-two states in the U.S., which it lists on its Web site. Each of these, in turn, makes resources (often including support groups) available to people in that state who seek information and support about TBI. Support groups help their participants by sharing knowledge, providing emotional support, and providing a place to network and learn from others who face similar circumstances.

There are even on-line resources available to take the place of in-person support groups for those who might find it difficult to participate in a face-to-face support group. The Brain Injury Association of America is listed as a partner of CaringBridge to help people with TBI, their family members, and their friends stay connected during a health crisis, treatment, and recovery. The free, non-profit CaringBridge Web service (www. caringbridge.org) allows TBI victims or their families to set up their own private, easily accessible Web site on which to share information and support. An excellent on-line resource is www.brainline.org, which characterizes itself as a resource devoted to preventing, treating, and living with traumatic brain injury. This multimedia collaborative project by public broadcaster WETA, funded by the Defense and Veterans Brain Injury Center, covers this issue for not only adults but also children. The Defense and Veterans Brain Injury Center (www.dvbic.org) itself has an informative Web site aimed at supporting traumatic brain injured military personnel and their families.

Another valuable source of information is http:// janetcromer.com/resources. Developed by Janet Cromer, RN, MA, LMHC, author of *Professor Cromer Learns to Read: A Couple's New Life after Brain Injury*, this Web site provides resources and links for brain injury survivors and their families and care-givers.

The pervasiveness of TBI has led to many books of advice being written for victims and families about living with brain injury. Among these are Garry Prowe, *Successfully Surviving a Brain Injury: A Family Guidebook, From the Emergency Room to Selecting a Rehabilitation Facility*, Brain Injury Success Books, 2010; John W. Cassidy and Lee Woodruff, *Mindstorms: Living with Traumatic Brain Injury*, Da Capo Lifelong Books, 2009; Richard C. Selenick and Karla Dougherty, *Living with Brain Injury: A Guide for Families*, Delmar Publishers, 2001; Ruthann K. Johansen, *Listening in the Silence, Seeing in the Dark: Reconstructing Life After Brain Injury*, Joseph Henry Press, 2002; Dorothy Gronwal, Philip Wrightson, and Peter Waddel, *Head Injury: The Facts:*

A Guide for Families and Care-givers, Oxford University Press, 1998; and Cheryle Sullivan, *Brain Injury Survival Kit: 365 Tips, Tools and Tricks to Deal with Cognitive Function Loss*, Demos Health, 2008.

The Traumatic Brain Injury Survival Guide, which is both a book and a Web site (www.tbiguide.com) maintained by a clinical neuropsychologist, offers practical advice in plain language on such topics as coping with common problems of TBI and dealing with physicians. It also addresses questions like how long the course of recovery might be, what to expect, and the functions and goals of the various professionals who might in any way be involved in treating a TBI victim.

If I may add a little personal advice for someone who has is recovering from a traumatic brain injury, advice based solely on Joanie's experience and not from the research or reading I have done, it would be this. As you recover, resume your former activities as soon as you are ready and comfortable to, but not before. People will ask you with more genuine concern than they might have before your TBI "How are you?" They may see you as a person with TBI, while you may feel less and less like one as time goes on. Be frank with them, telling them you're back 100% to where you were before, or you still have some trouble finding words, or you still have difficulty following conversations, or everything's fine except your reading has slowed down, or whatever it may be. There's no gain in telling them that everything is now fine with you if it is not, or, conversely, that you are not fully recovered when you are. Do your rehabilitation exercises diligently to speed your recovery. Be patient: everything in recovery takes more time, and every improvement happens more slowly, than you might expect. You may find yourself reaching a plateau in your recovery. Courage, though, for it may only be a plateau and not necessarily the summit. Deal with it, but don't dwell on it. Keep on stepping. Keep yourself safe. Keep yourself healthy.

Joanie's experience showed me that those who have to deal with TBI, both its sufferers and their families, face a tough battle. But it also showed me that it can be survived by many and that many of its victims can fight their way back to where they were before. As a community, we need to devote the necessary resources and effort to improve our understanding of how to prevent traumatic brain injuries, treat them when they occur, and provide for the extensive rehabilitation that its victims may require in order to return to their former levels of functioning. We need to be more aware of this silent epidemic and do a better job of combating it.

SOURCES

⚜

A NUMBER OF SOURCES provided the information about traumatic brain injury, health care delivery, and other factual matters discussed in this book.

Chapter 2

Information about the characteristics of subdural hematoma and traumatic brain injury is from Brain Injury Association of America's Web site, "Living with Brain Injury," http://www.biausa.org/living-with-brain-injury.htm [accessed January 13, 2011] and from the National Institute of Neurological Disorders and Stroke, "NINDS Traumatic Brain Injury Information Page," http://www.ninds.nih.gov/disorders/tbi/tbi.htm [accessed January 13, 2011].

Chapter 3

The brief history of Maynard, Massachusetts is taken in part from http://web.maynard.ma.us/history/mill-history.htm [accessed January 13, 2011].

Chapter 5

The quotation about the perforator used to drill into skull bone is from Katrina Firlik's book *Another Day in the Frontal Lobe*. New York: Random House, 2007: p. 96.

Afterword

Dr. William Brody's characterization of the U.S. health care system as the industrial world's most inefficient medical system is reported in an article by Maria Blackburn, "Bright Ideas." *Johns Hopkins Magazine* 60, no.1 (February 2008): p. 41. The problems with the U.S. health care system discussed in this chapter are enumerated by the American College of Physicians in "Achieving a High-Performance Health Care System with Universal Access: What the United States Can Learn from Other Countries." *Annals of Internal Medicine* 148, no. 1 (January 2008).

The description of the hospitalist specialty as it was just beginning to make its mark in the 1990s is from an article by Christopher P. Noel, "The Emerging Role of the Hospitalist." *Physicians News Digest* (February 1998): p. 298. The growth of the hospitalist movement since that time is described in Niraj Sehgal and Robert M. Wachter, "The Expanding Role of Hospitalists in the United States." *Medicine Weekly* 136 (2006): pp. 591-596.

Jeffrey Krasner's article in *The Boston Globe Magazine*, March 8, 2009 (© Copyright 2009, Globe Newspaper

Company, Inc.), is the source of the cogent quotes on case management.

The letter quoted by the Harvard researcher is Jo M. Solet, "Hospitals, Don't Turn up the Volume, Lower the Noise." *Boston Sunday Globe*, February 28, 2010: p. C8. The trial efforts aimed at reducing noise instituted at several hospitals are described in: Anonymous, "Researchers Find Ways to Reduce Noise in Hospitals." *Association of Operating Room Nurses. AORN Journal.* 83 (2006), no. 1: p. 74; Patricia R. Johnson and Lisa Thornhill, "Noise Reduction in the Hospital Setting." *Journal of Nursing Care Quality* 21 (2006), no. 4: p. 295; "Enhance the Healing Environment by Reducing Noise." *Environment of Care News* 8 (June 2005): pp. 10-11; and "Fixing the Noisy Hospital." *Boston Sunday Globe*, May 30, 2010: pp. C1, C3. Current standards for health care facility design and construction can be found in Facilities Guidelines Institute, *Guidelines for Design and Construction of Health Care Facilities*, 2010 Edition.

The discussion of the epidemiology of traumatic brain injury is a compilation of information from a number of sources: "How Many People Have TBI?" Centers for Disease Control and Prevention http://www.cdc.gov/traumaticbraininjury/statistics.html [accessed January 24, 2011]; Jean A. Langlois, Wesley Rutland-Brown, and Karen E. Thomas, *Traumatic Brain Injury in the United States: Emergency Department Visits, Hospitalizations, and Deaths* 2002-2006. Atlanta, GA:

Centers for Disease Control and Prevention, National Center for Injury Prevention and Control, 2006; D. J. Thurman, C. Alverson, K. Dunn, J. Guerrero, and J. E. Sniezek, "Traumatic Brain Injury in the United States: A Public Health Perspective." *Journal of Head Trauma Rehabilitation* 14, no. 6, (1999): pp. 602–615; and William J. Winslade, *Confronting Traumatic Brain Injury: Devastation, Hope and Healing*. New Haven: Yale University Press, 1998.

Several authorities have used the term "silent epidemic" to characterize the general lack of awareness among the population at large of the incidence and prevalence of traumatic brain injury, among them Michael Fraas and Margaret Calvert, "Stories From a 'Silent Epidemic:' Oral History Project Counters Myths about Traumatic Brain Injury." *The ASHA Leader* 11, no. 15, (2006): pp. 10-11, 30; and the University of Pennsylvania's Center for Brain Injury and Repair http://www.med.upenn.edu/cbir/silent_epidemic [accessed January 13, 2011].

The detailed description of the types of traumatic brain injury and their symptoms is abstracted from the National Institute of Neurological Disorders and Stroke's "Brain Injury Information Page," September 15, 2008.

The quotation "Most traumatic brain injuries shatter more than one life" is from William J. Winslade,

Confronting Traumatic Brain Injury: Devastation, Hope and Healing. New Haven: Yale University Press, 1998: p. 92.

Several sources provide the basis for the discussion of head injuries resulting from playing sports: Seth Mnookin, "When to Hang It Up." *The Boston Globe Magazine* (May 6, 2007): pp. 29-31, 40-44; Alan Schwarz, "New Sign of Brain Damage in N.F.L." *The New York Times* (January 28, 2009): p. B11; and Christopher Nowinski, *Head Games: Football's Concussion Crisis from the NFL to Youth Leagues*. East Bridgewater, MA: Drummond Publishing Group, 2007.

The National Safety Council is the source of statistics about child seat belt use; see "The Evidence Is In: Adults Who Don't Buckle Up Have a Dangerous Impact on Children's Safety," http://www.nsc.org/airbag.aspx [accessed May 20, 2007].

The recommendation for hallway lighting is from Walecia Konrad, "Make Room for Mom(s)." *Money* 36, no. 7 (July 2007): pp. 49-51.

ACKNOWLEDGMENTS

There are many people to thank for their support of Joanie and me during the troubling journey described in this book and, afterward, for their help in getting this book published. Here they are, and if I've forgotten anyone, I hope you will forgive me.

Todd and Janna Kerpelman, our children, rushed to our sides after Joanie's accident and gave us both their love, strength, and support to help us through this crisis. All the friends, neighbors, and relatives who plied us with food, flowers, cards, and, most of all, concern and caring during Joanie's hospitalizations and recovery were of immeasurable help. To all the regulars at "the Bean," and especially Boston Bean House's owners, Dawn and Eli Schallhorn, for providing the kind of community that Joan and I are so glad to be a part of and that gave Joan a place of retreat to strive to return to, thank you for your support.

Joanie and I are indebted to the health care and rehabilitation professionals who helped bring her back to normal functioning after her traumatic brain injury. To the staffs of Emerson Hospital, the Lahey Clinic, and Emerson Hospital Home Care for providing supportive, compassionate care, Joanie and I give our heartfelt thanks.

We especially thank the physicians and nurses of the neurosurgical team at Lahey Clinic Hospital who treated her, Dr. John Halporn for caring for and about Joanie even when she was no longer formally in his care, and Mary Ann Butler for her persistence and skill in helping Joanie recover her cognitive functioning.

My friends Bob Runck, Dave Didriksen, owner of Willow Books of Acton, Manya Chylinski, president of Alley 424 Communications in Boston, Dan Edson, Linda Watskin, and Janet Cromer, author of *Professor Cromer Learns to Read: A Couple's New Life After Brain Injury*, gave me helpful advice about publishing this book.

Thanks go to writing colleagues who helped me polish my writing along the way: the participants of the Maynard writing group, led by Linda Watskin, and those at a number of workshops and seminars at Grub Street Writers in Boston.

Several people read and critiqued parts of early drafts of this book, including my children Todd and Janna, Dr. Geoffrey Kurland, Medical Director of Pediatric Heart and Lung Transplantation at the University of Pittsburgh School of Medicine and author of *My Own Medicine: A Doctor's Life as a Patient*, and my writing friends Nichole Bernier, author of *The Unfinished*

Work of Elizabeth D, and Meg Larson. I am especially indebted to several others who, in addition to my wife, committed to read all of a later draft of this book and provide me with comments on how to improve it. They are Tanja Crumley, of the American Diabetes Association, Dr. Jo M. Solet, Instructor in Medicine at Cambridge Health Alliance and Harvard Medical School, Dr. Henry Vaillant, Chair of the Department of Medicine at Emerson Hospital, and Linda Watskin. Their critical insights improved the accuracy of this book's contents and the narrative flow of my writing. Any errors or omissions of either style or substance are mine, however, not theirs.

About the Author

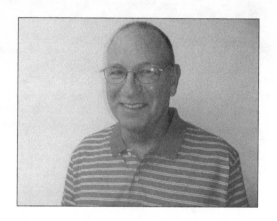

An award-winning health care writer and editor, Larry C. Kerpelman, Ph.D. has published two academic books and written numerous articles for publications such as *The Journal of the American Medical Association*, *The Chronicle of Higher Education*, *The Boston Globe*, and *GreenPrints* magazine. His bachelor's degree in psychology is from the Johns Hopkins University, and his doctorate in clinical psychology is from the University of Rochester. His four-decade-long professional career spanned research, teaching, and consulting in human behavior and in public policy issues. He lives in Acton, Massachusetts, with his wife Joanie and spends his time writing, traveling, volunteering, and walking to his favorite coffee house.

Visit the author's Web site at

www.LCKerpelman.com

to learn more.